THE FACTS ABOUT HEADACHE

DID YOU KNOW . . .

- Between 50 and 70 million Americans have recurring headaches: migraines, tension headaches, cluster headaches, and more.

- Many common foods such as cheese, nuts, and baked goods can trigger severe headaches.

- You can fight back against headache pain WITHOUT DRUGS.

- Each headache leaves clues behind. you can use the ~~separate~~ and ~~there~~ ~~make~~ this book to find out ~~and~~ ~~how~~ ~~minimize~~ or

—find inside

THE DELL MEDICAL LIBRARY

Relief from Chronic Backache
Relief from Chronic Headache
Relief from Chronic TMJ Pain
Relief from Chronic Arthritis Pain
Learning to Live with Chronic IBS
Learning to Live with Chronic Fatigue Syndrome

THE DELL MEDICAL LIBRARY

Relief from

CHRONIC HEADACHE

Antonia van der Meer

Foreword by Seymour Diamond, M.D.

A LYNN SONBERG BOOK

Published by
Dell Publishing
a division of
Bantam Doubleday Dell Publishing Group, Inc.
666 Fifth Avenue
New York, New York 10103

Published by arrangement with Lynn Sonberg Book Services,
166 East 56 Street, New York, New York 10022

ISBN: 0-440-20570-0

Printed in the United States of America
Published simultaneously in Canada

June 1990

10 9 8 7 6 5 4 3 2 1

OPM

CONTENTS

Important Note: Medical science and headache research are constantly evolving and subject to reinterpretation. Although every effort has been made to include the most up-to-date and accurate information in this book, there can be no guarantee that this information won't change with time and further research. Furthermore, because of the large number of conditions, problems, and studies that are directly or indirectly related to headaches (an estimated three hundred conditions can cause headaches), it is impossible to include everything in this basic guide to headaches. The reader should bear in mind that this book is not to be used for the purpose of self-diagnosis or self-treatment and that any and all medical problems should be referred to the expertise of the appropriate medical personnel.

ACKNOWLEDGMENTS

Thanks to the following for their time, expertise, information, and advice:

Dr. Seymour Diamond, director of the Diamond Headache Clinic, Chicago, Illinois, and Executive Director, National Headache Foundation

Dr. Ninan Mathew, director of the Houston Headache Clinic, Houston, Texas

Dr. Paul S. Silver, Ph.D., assistant clinical professor of psychiatry and psychology at the University of Texas Southwest Medical School at Dallas

Linda Barbanel, M.S.W., C.S.W., Manhattan psychotherapist

Dr. Ajax George, senior neuroradiologist, New York University Medical Center, and Professor of Radiology at NYU Medical School

The National Headache Foundation, Chicago, Illinois

The American Association for the Study of Headaches, San Clemente, California

FOREWORD

Every year, over 45 million Americans seek medical help for headaches. Frequently, physicians provide patients with diagnoses, but physicians aren't always the best sources of information about what patients can do on their own to minimize their headache pain.

Many others who experience headaches never seek medical help at all because they are afraid that some potentially catastrophic condition such as a brain tumor or an aneurysm is the cause of their problem. Fortunately, their fears are rarely warranted, as the vast majority of headache problems do not arise from underlying disease. The good news is that nearly all headaches can be controlled and treated.

This excellent book, *Relief from Chronic Headache,* by Antonia van der Meer, enables headache sufferers to identify the type of headache they are experiencing and learn about the treatment methods available. The reassuring text succeeds in providing practical information and guidance in dealing with headaches. The various chapters focus on the different types of headaches, including migraine, cluster, tension, organic, and miscellaneous headaches. A discussion of the importance of "headache education" is included. The author also faces the challenge of "diagnostic dilemmas" in an interesting and thorough approach.

The headache sufferer is presented with a variety of interventions that can be utilized in preventing headaches. Self-help and coping skills are discussed. A variety of nondrug therapies—such as diet, biofeedback, relaxation training, and other methods that can be self-administered by the patient—are explored; they are all helpful adjuncts in coping with a chronic headache problem. One especially useful chapter provides information on how and where to find help for headaches and a list of headache clinics throughout the United States.

Some headache sufferers experience psychological problems that existed prior to the onset of the headache disorder and that may contribute to the headache problem. Other patients may experience psychological problems that are secondary to the chronic headache. Enhancing a patient's knowledge about psychological problems may be a vital factor in alleviating chronic headaches.

I found this book to be extremely enjoyable and informative. For the past thirty-five years I have been involved in the treatment of headaches, and I currently serve as executive director of the National Headache Foundation. As director of the Chicago-based Diamond Headache Clinic, I have had the advantage of personally observing thousands of headache sufferers and can fully understand the difficulties they face. Many headache sufferers spend endless hours searching for information about their problem and undergo years of worthless therapies, testing, and suffering without ever finding relief. Educating patients that they themselves can play a vital role in preventing and relieving their headaches is essential. New modes of treatment are available. This text offers the reader an excellent resource for finding information about the causes of and therapies for headache. It also discusses the extensive research being conducted into the causes and treatment of chronic headache. I would highly recommend it to my patients and their families.

As this book makes clear, headache victims do not have to suffer in silence. By learning to help themselves, they can find much-needed relief from pain as they regain control of their lives.

SEYMOUR DIAMOND, M.D.
Executive Director
National Headache Foundation

INTRODUCTION

This book is for you if you are one of the millions of headache sufferers in the United States who want to regain control of their lives and stop the pain that plagues them. You don't have to suffer quietly any longer. In buying this book, you have taken the first step in getting on with your life. You bought it because you want to know more about the pain that touches your everyday life and you want to find ways to control it.

This book describes the physiology of headache pain and takes you through various diagnostic processes that can help you pinpoint the type of headache you most frequently have. You'll learn about tension headaches, migraines, cluster headaches, and others. There's a headache diary to be completed that will enable you to take a look at the way headaches affect you—how often they hit you, how long they last, and what circumstances aggravate them. You'll find out about many nondrug methods that you can use to fight headache pain *now*. You'll also find out where to find help if you need to seek medical care and what to expect of your doctors.

There are many techniques that can help you prevent headaches. However, even if you are unable to prevent them, this book can also help you find ways to cope with the pain itself. Last but not least, this book discusses the psychological effects of headaches—the way sufferers and their families relate, how some people try to deny their chronic headache pain, and more. With the help of this book, you can reclaim your life and, it is hoped, suffer fewer headaches than you did in the past.

ONE

HEAD OF THE CLASS— AN EDUCATION IN HEADACHES

One of the most common—and most distressing—of all medical complaints is the headache. Although the medical community knows a great deal about the causes of and treatments for headaches, we are still a long way from understanding all the mysteries of the inner workings of the brain. One thing we can be sure of, however, is that headache sufferers are not alone in their misery. The ailment is, in fact, almost universal; very few people have never had a headache.

For most people, a headache is a passing annoyance. But for many others, headaches are severe, chronic, and even incapacitating. Headaches are not visible to other people, and for this reason other people may insist that chronic headache sufferers' pain is "all in their heads." Although it is sometimes extremely difficult to diagnose the precise cause of a headache, be assured—the pain you feel is definitely real.

If you are a headache sufferer, take heart. There is hope, and there is help. You are one of a large group of sufferers who are also looking for ways to cope with the realities of their headaches.

A few interesting facts will give you a sample of what we do know about headaches.

- Each year in the United States, headaches account for 80 million doctor appointments.

- American headache sufferers collectively lose 157 million workdays a year.

- Over 45 million Americans experience recurring headaches.

- Women are twice as likely to experience chronic headache pain as men.

- An estimated 18 million Americans get migraines.

- An estimated 50 million pounds of aspirin is taken every year for headache relief.

- Each year, Americans spend some $400 million on over-the-counter pain relievers.

- In 1987, the National Institutes of Health spent $932,000 on headache research.

- Less than 10 percent of all headaches are caused by an underlying disease such as sinus infection, glaucoma, temporomandibular joint disorder (TMJ), or tumor.

- Famous people who suffered from headaches include Julius Caesar, Lewis Carroll, Frédéric Chopin, Charles Darwin, Sigmund Freud, Thomas Jefferson, Edgar Allan Poe, and Virginia Woolf.

- Headaches predate recorded history. Skeletons of prehistoric humans have been found with holes drilled into the skull—perhaps a method of relieving headache pain. This certainly seems a horrific and barbaric alternative to aspirin, but it is interesting to note that small holes are still occasionally drilled in the skull today as a neurosurgical approach to relieve abnormally high pressure levels in the skull.

WHAT IS A HEADACHE?

Quite simply, a headache is a pain in the head, face, or neck. The pain may be a throbbing, aching, stabbing, or burning sensation.

The causes of headaches are much debated. Only fifty years ago, migraine was thought to be a psychosomatic disorder, and migraine sufferers were looked upon with skepticism. Then scientists discovered that headaches are caused by muscular tension, by pathological problems, or by vascular changes (the dilation and constriction of blood vessels) in the head.

Today, doctors and scientists believe there may be more to it than this. The discomfort caused by blood vessels and muscles may be only a symptom of a biological abnormality in the brain and nerves. People with chronic headaches, especially migraines, may be predisposed to them because of abnormalities in the actions of certain brain chemicals.

Serotonin is a brain chemical linked to headache. It acts as a messenger and influences sleep, mood, and the constriction and dilation of blood vessels. If serotonin resources are depleted, a migraine headache may result. Occasionally, the amount of serotonin is not itself the problem; rather, certain enzymes may be destroying serotonin and depleting serotonin levels. Or receptors or depots that normally receive or release serotonin may be defective and may not receive or release enough of the chemical into the system. Physicians are identifying different types of receptors or depots, and research is concentrating on how they influence migraines.

Headache research is also focusing on serotonin levels in the brain and on what factors affect those levels. But the actual physiological cause of headaches remains somewhat unclear. Basically, we know that muscular, pathological, and vascular changes cause pain, and that these changes may or may not be influenced by certain brain chemical changes. But the external factors that seem to provoke headaches are better documented than the physiological factors.

TYPES OF HEADACHE

Not all headaches are created equal. Some are mild, and some are severe. Some are the result of stress or hunger; others are connected to a disease or an ongoing problem such as arthritis. What follows is a listing and brief description of a variety of headaches. Some of these headaches are discussed in more depth in later chapters. Only your doctor can tell you which type of headache you actually suffer from, but this listing will introduce you to the array of headache types and offers initial clues about which type is most likely plaguing you.

Tension Headache

The tension headache is perhaps the most common headache. It results from tightness in the head and neck muscles. A tension headache feels like a generalized ache or viselike pain rather than throbbing or pounding. It is not related to any underlying diseases. Tension headaches may be either acute (episodic) or chronic (recurrent). Acute tension headaches can result from a recent episode of stress or fatigue. Chronic tension headaches may be the result of deeply rooted depression or other psychological difficulties.

Hypertension Headache

Hypertension headaches are found in people with high blood pressure. They are usually most severe in the morning, and the pain wears off as the day goes on. The pressure either is generalized or forms a "hatband" around the head.

Migraine Headache

A vascular headache (that is, a headache related to blood vessel dilation), the migraine's symptoms are not limited to head pain. Attacks may also include nausea, vomiting, dizziness, numbness, and visual disturbances. They usually strike only one side of the head or one specific location, such as an eye or a temple. (In fact, the word *migraine* comes from the Greek word *hemicrania,* which means "an ailment of half the head." In Old English, *migraine* was *megrim.*) No one clearly understands the cause of migraines, but they are quite a common affliction. Women make up 75 percent of migraine sufferers. The tendency to have migraines seems to be inherited—the great majority of migraine sufferers have family members who also suffer from migraines.

Cluster Headache

Cluster headaches usually strike men, who make up 90 percent of sufferers. The pain is extremely severe and has been known to drive patients to bang their heads against walls or even to contemplate suicide. Most victims of cluster headaches are smokers. Like migraines, cluster headaches are localized, tending to affect only one part of the head. They may be limited to the eye area only. The intensity and type of pain, however, is different from that of migraines—it may be a searing, boring pain or an excruciating throbbing. The nose becomes congested or runny on one side of the face. One eye may become bloodshot and teary. Cluster headaches may last only twenty minutes, but they can recur many times in one day and every day for weeks. Sufferers may then be headache free for months or even years afterward, only to experience another bout of cluster headaches later. There are no preliminary symptoms that warn a person that he is about to get a cluster headache.

Menstrual Headache

The pain of a menstrual headache is migrainelike. It occurs on or after the onset of ovulation and disappears at or during the period. The regular monthly occurrence of a woman's headaches is the most important indicator of a menstrual headache.

Exertion Headache

An exertion headache starts after some type of physical exertion, possibly including sex. For some people, coughing or laughing can bring on an exertion headache. About 10 percent of exertion headache sufferers are actually suffering from a separate physical ailment, such as a tumor or a brain aneurysm (weakened blood vessel) and should see a doctor right away.

Sinus Headache

Sinus headaches are caused by a clogged sinus cavity that is unable to drain due to infection.

Temporal Arteritis

Affecting mostly people aged fifty and over, the temporal arteritis headache is caused by inflamed arteries in the head and neck. The pain is a burning or jabbing sensation. Temporal arteritis is a rare but potentially serious problem that may lead to stroke or blindness. It requires prompt treatment.

TMJ Headache

Temporomandibular joint disorder is a problem with the jaw joint (where the lower jaw meets the skull) and its muscles. It may be caused by misaligned teeth, jaw clenching, or teeth grinding and is thought to affect as many as 10 million Americans. TMJ may cause a variety of symptoms and pain. Headaches are quite commonly one result.

Hangover Headache

A hangover headache is linked to the consumption of alcohol, which dilates and irritates the brain's blood vessels and surrounding tissue. The throbbing pain resembles that of a migraine. Hangover headaches are often accompanied by feelings of nausea.

Allergy Headache

The onset of an allergy headache is heralded by watery eyes and nasal congestion. The allergy that causes these headaches is usually seasonal, such as a pollen allergy, and not a food allergy.

Caffeine Withdrawal Headache

Caffeine, a substance found in many foods and drinks, constricts the blood vessels. Many people who skip their customary cup of coffee in the morning or who don't drink any caffeinated beverages on weekends suffer from a caffeine withdrawal headache. It is caused by a boomerang effect of the blood vessels, which dilate in response to the lack of caffeine. The dilation causes the headache pain.

Tic Douloureux

Tic douloureux is a relatively rare disease of the neural impulses that is most often found in women over the age of fifty-five. Sufferers experience short, jablike pains in the face and should seek medical attention right away.

Tumor Headache

While almost everyone who gets a headache immediately suspects that it may be the sign of a brain tumor, it is only rarely actually so. Only between 0.1 and 0.5 percent of headache patients have previously undetected brain tumors. Symptoms of a tumor headache include pain that worsens, often coupled with projectile vomiting, speech and vision disturbances, coordination or balance problems, and seizures.

Other Headaches

Other types of headaches that plague people are related to trauma, hunger, fever, arthritis, and eyestrain. A *trauma headache* (caused by a blow to the head) may appear to be a migraine, but it persists daily and is resistant to treatment. *Hunger headaches* strike around mealtime, when blood sugar is low and a rebound dilation of the blood vessels takes place. A *fever headache* is the result of an inflammation of the blood vessels in the head. *Arthritis* can be at the root of headache pain because of an inflammation of the joints and muscles in the head or neck. The pain intensifies with movement. *Eyestrain headaches* usually cause aching at the front of the head and are related to vision problems such as astigmatism.

PAIN PERCEPTION

The brain itself is relatively insensitive to pain, but the coverings of the brain—including the membranes, arteries, and nerves—can feel pain. The amount of pain a headache sufferer feels depends not only on the severity of the headache itself but also on how the person perceives and reacts to pain, known as the *pain threshold*.

No two people have the same pain threshold. A person's pain threshold may change during his or her life, depending on psychological and physical factors. In general, happiness and well-being tend to make people more resistant to pain, while depression lowers their pain threshold. Lower pain thresholds during periods of depression may be due to lowered levels of endorphins in the body. Endorphins are substances manufactured in the brain that have pain-killing properties.

MEDICAL ATTENTION

Not every headache should send you running for a doctor. If your headaches are more than a passing nuisance, however, you will probably want to discuss them with a physician. There are many headaches that do demand medical attention.

You should never feel embarrassed about seeking medical help for a health issue of concern to you. There's no reason to suffer just because you assume your headache is not "life threatening." In general, you should see a doctor whenever you feel that your headaches are frequent enough or bothersome enough to warrant a visit.

Medical attention is a must if you experience any of the following headaches:

• A sudden, extremely severe headache that differs from your usual headache pattern. (This is occasionally a symptom of a brain aneurysm.)

- A headache that becomes continuous and builds in severity. (This may—albeit rarely—be a sign of a tumor.)

- Headaches that increase in frequency.

- A headache that is coupled with neurological symptoms, including weakness of limbs, numbness, or visual disturbances.

- A headache that is coupled with fever, sore throat, shortness of breath, or symptoms of the ear or nose. (This could point to anything from meningitis to heart disease.)

- Headaches that begin after age fifty-five. (This may be a sign of temporal arteritis, tic douloureux, or other serious disease.)

- A headache caused by a head injury, especially if accompanied by confusion, slurred speech, numbness, fever, or clear fluid or blood running from the nose or ears.

- A headache that involves eye or ear pain.

- A headache that is experienced for the first time by a child.

- Headaches that do not respond to treatment.

- A debilitating headache.

- Headaches that interfere with your relationships, your work, or your life.

- Changes in the character of the headache.

- Headaches that cause you to take over-the-counter pain medications on a daily basis.

Go immediately to an emergency room if you suspect a ruptured aneurysm, or stroke (unbearable pain combined with stiff neck, double vision, and possible loss of consciousness), or meningitis (a headache accompanied by fever, joint pain, and sore throat), or if you have had a serious head injury.

DETERMINING YOUR HEADACHE TYPE

When you read through the various headache types, you may have noticed that some resembled your headaches and were even surprisingly like the headaches you get, while others didn't resemble yours at all. You probably ruled out many of the headache types immediately as not pertaining to you. In the next chapter you will have a chance to fill out a headache diary, which may bring you closer to determining the type of headache you suffer from. Once you have completed the diary, you will have many more clues as to why, how, and when you suffer headache pain. Refer back to this chapter then to see if you can spot your headache type.

THE COMPLETE
HEADACHE DIARY

As a headache sufferer, your first step in taking charge of your health is to learn as much as you can about when and why the pain strikes. Before you read any further, it's important to document your headaches. Identifying the type and intensity of your headaches, as well as their warning signs and symptoms, can help you and your doctor develop a treatment program or plan. *Please remember that only your doctor can make a diagnosis.* The purpose of this diary is simply to reveal some of the possible connections and patterns in your headaches.

Try to be honest and faithful to this diary. Record all pertinent facts, and stick with it for at least a month. Use the "Comments" section to catalog any precipitating factors that you think may trigger your headaches. A pattern may begin to emerge; your headaches may seem to be tied to a certain time of the month, to work stress, to weekend sleep patterns, or even to your consumption of caffeine.

Here's how to use the diary:

1. Photocopy the diary pages on pages 17–20, or use a blank notebook with the columns labeled as specified (date, warning signs, and the rest).

2. Every time you experience headache pain, fill in all the pertinent information in the diary. The first entry has been filled in as an example for you to follow.
3. Keep the diary for at least a month.
4. Using your completed diary entries, fill in the "Headache Diary Analysis." Try to discover any patterns or regularities in your headaches.
5. If your headaches strike infrequently or if no pattern emerges, continue the diary for another month. Fill out the "Headache Diary Analysis" once again.
6. Bring the diary and analysis with you to your doctor if you seek medical help for your headaches. It may prove helpful in diagnosing and treating you.

HEADACHE DIARY

Example:

Date	11/5
Warning signs	hunger
Time begun	2:30
Time ended	8 P.M.
Type of pain	throb
Intensity of pain	1 2 3 4 ⑤ 6 7 8 9
Location	forehead
Treatment or medication taken	none
Effect of treatment	n/a
Comments	skipped lunch, under pressure at work

Date _____

Warning signs _____

Time begun _____

Time ended _____

Type of pain _____

Intensity of pain   1 2 3 4 5 6 7 8 9

Location _____

Treatment or
medication taken _____

Effect of treatment _____

Comments _____

Date _____

Warning signs _____

Time begun _____

Time ended _____

Type of pain _____

Intensity of pain   1 2 3 4 5 6 7 8 9

Location _____

Treatment or
medication taken _____

Effect of treatment _____

Comments _____

Date   _____

Warning signs   _____

Time begun   _____

Time ended   _____

Type of pain   _____

Intensity of pain   1 2 3 4 5 6 7 8 9

Location   _____

Treatment or
medication taken   _____

Effect of treatment   _____

Comments   _____

HEADACHE DIARY ANALYSIS

Personal History

Sex _____

Age _____

Weight _____

Exercise plan, if any _____

Age when you can first remember getting headaches _____

Other family members, if any, who suffer from headaches

_____

_____

_____

Headache Summary

Total number of headaches in one week _____

Total number of headaches in one month _____

Number of morning headaches _____

Number of afternoon headaches _____

Number of all-day or multiday headaches _____

Number of headaches affecting the whole head _____

Number of headaches affecting only one side or a portion of the head _____

Were any of your headaches debilitating? YES   NO

If so, how many? _____

Number of headaches that were mild to moderately intense _____

Do any of your headaches awaken you at night? YES   NO

Do any of your headaches awaken you early in the morning? YES   NO

Do any of your headaches prevent you from falling asleep at night? YES   NO

Average duration of headache (minutes or hours) _____

Average pain intensity of headache: 1 2 3 4 5 6 7 8 9

In the "Comments" sections, you have recorded things that you think may have triggered your headaches. Check the number of headaches that you think were triggered by:

Emotional stress (family fights, work worries, etc.) _____

Oversleeping or change in sleep schedule (from weekday to weekend) _____

Lack of sleep _____

Exercise or overexertion _____

Foods eaten (Chinese food, hard cheese, chocolate) _____

Fasting, skipped meals, or delayed meals _____

Premenstrual syndrome _____

Change in status quo (job, house, or routine) _____

Crisis (divorce, death, etc.) _____

Change in the weather _____

Physical illness _____

Fatigue _____

Other _____

Treatment Summary

Number of times you took a pain reliever for a headache _____

List all the treatments that you tried (aspirin, massage, food avoidance, prescription drugs, etc.)

_____

_____

_____

Which, if any, of these treatments helped you cope with or relieve the pain?

_____

_____

Did any of the treatments you tried make the pain worse? YES NO
If so, which? _____

Headache-Free Period Summary

Take a moment to reflect on your headache-free days, weeks, or months. What was happening at work and at home during these times? What types of foods were you eating or not eating? Were your bedtime or napping schedules different? If you are a woman, at what point in your menstrual cycle were you headache free? Write your comments and perceptions here.

_____

_____

_____

_____

_____

After you complete your headache diary, you should have a clearer idea of your headache type and what factors trigger your pain. Once the precipitating factors are pinpointed, you may be able to avoid them. For example, if you realize that your headaches are being caused by foods, you can modify your diet. This is an important first step in learning how to control your headaches.

The more you and your doctor know about your headaches, the easier diagnosis and treatment will be. If, after completing the diary, you suspect that you have a specific headache type, turn to the corresponding chapter or section and learn more about the physiological details of—and treatment for—that type of headache.

THREE

MIGRAINES

Migraine headaches can be devastating, but you needn't feel resigned to living with them. By finding out as much as you can about them, by paying attention to the factors that seem to trigger them, and by reading in this chapter about the treatments available, you can gain control of headaches that today seem to be controlling you.

Although people have known about migraines for thousands of years, medical science is a long way from fully understanding the syndrome. Even as late as the 1950s, headache books still listed migraines under epilepsy. Later, migraines were thought to be a psychosomatic disorder. Today we know that migraines are vascular headaches, brought on by changes in the blood vessels in the head. We also know that migraines can strike almost anyone with pain that is very real and very unpleasant.

A person's first migraine attack can occur anytime between the ages of five and forty, but most first migraines occur during the teen years. If you are going to suffer from migraines, you will almost certainly have had one before the age of forty. Males and females are affected about equally by migraines during puberty, but later in life there is a predominance of women sufferers. The tendency to get migraines seems to run in families. Between 70 and 90 percent of migraine patients report having other migraine sufferers in their families, suggesting that susceptibility to migraine is hereditary. According to the National Headache Foundation, the actual breakdown is as follows: If both parents get migraines, there is a 75 percent chance of their child getting them. If only one parent experiences migraines, then the child's chance drops to 50 percent. If a distant relative suffers from migraines, offspring have a 20 percent chance of developing migraines.

Migraine strikes as many as 18 million people. Attacks can range from moderate to quite severe. They may be infrequent or frequent, sometimes occurring as often as weekly. They usually affect only one side of the head, but they strike both sides in some people. There are two types: the classic migraine and the common migraine.

The *classic migraine* has a noticeable preheadache phase that warns the person that an attack is imminent. The preheadache phase is also called the *prodromal phase* or the *aura*. For many people, this phase is the most frightening part of the attack. It is thought to be the result of constricting blood vessels, which reduces the blood flow to the brain. During the prodromal phase, there may be visual disturbances, speech disorders, numbness, sweating, tingling in the face, weakness in an arm or leg, or other signs. Visual disturbances may include *scotomata* (blind spots) or *fortification spectrum* (a zigzag pattern). Flashing lights may also be seen. Figures may be distorted, à la *Alice in Wonderland*. Speech disorders most often include difficulty finding the right word. Very rarely, the sufferer finds he cannot speak at all.

Some sufferers experience this preheadache phase without getting the subsequent headache. More commonly, however, the preheadache constriction of the blood vessels is followed by a dilation of the blood vessels ten to thirty minutes later, causing a pounding, throbbing pain. These changes in the blood vessels are believed to be caused by brain chemistry changes. The pounding headache pain is often exacerbated by nausea, fatigue, irritability, vomiting, photophobia (sensitivity to light), phonophobia (sensitivity to sound), and rarely, constipation or diarrhea.

The *common migraine*, true to its name, is more common. Eighty percent of migraine sufferers experience common migraine. There is no preheadache phase or warning sign prior to the onset of pain in the common migraine. The throbbing, pounding pain of the common migraine is exactly the same as that of the headache phase of the classic migraine; the only difference between them is in what comes before.

Children can also get migraines. In fact, migraine often begins during the childhood years. In children, however, the actual headache portion of the migraine is often less pronounced than the nausea, vomiting, fever, and sensitivity to light. It may sometimes be difficult to diagnose these complaints, and the problem may at first be thought to be a stomach or intestinal disorder or even appendicitis.

Many people feel that children who get migraines have a certain personality—the "driven" personality, similar to the personality commonly associated with adult sufferers. Children, like adults, can become anxious about their work and social lives. Schoolwork can cause a lot of stress, as can switching schools, moving to a new town, or not getting invited to the right party.

Treatment for children is usually attempted without drugs. Children's headaches may be controlled through diet, good sleep and exercise habits, and the relaxation techniques of biofeedback. For a headache in progress, acetaminophen is usually offered. If the headaches become more severe or more frequent, physicians usually prescribe a prescription drug for the pain and nausea. The same drugs that are given to adults are given to children, but in smaller doses and strengths.

TIP-OFFS THAT YOU MAY SUFFER FROM MIGRAINES

Check the list of migraine headache symptoms below.

- Before the actual headache, you may experience an aura—a bizarre type of warning signal, such as a visual or speech disturbance, numbness, or even vertigo (dizziness).

- The headache is usually limited to one side of the head but may switch sides during the attack. (About one-third of sufferers find that both sides of the head pound.)

- The headache occurs from time to time but not every day.

- The pain is violent throbbing or pounding.

- The headache may be accompanied by nausea or vomiting.

- During the headache, you are extremely sensitive to light (photophobia).

- During the headache, you are extremely sensitive to sound (phonophobia). Even the ticking of a watch can be unbearable.

- During the headache, you prefer to lie still and try not to move your head. Head movement during an attack is painful.

- After the headache ends, you may experience a postheadache phase, during which you feel drained. The head may feel tender to the touch.

- The headache often occurs after a particularly stressful time.

- If you are a woman, the headache attacks may occur on a regular monthly basis, during ovulation or before menstruation.

- Certain foods and drinks, such as chocolate or alcohol, can set off the headache.

- Pressing on the affected temple or holding the affected side of the head may assuage the pain.

- The headache may last only a few hours, but the most common duration is from eight to twenty-four hours.

- The face may become pale; the hands and feet may become cold.

The migraine headache does not always follow the average textbook example. For this reason we strongly urge that you consult a doctor about any severe headaches or related illnesses. The signs and symptoms of migraines listed above are very general in nature. Only a medical doctor can make a reliable diagnosis.

THE MIGRAINE PERSONALITY

Who is most likely to suffer from migraine? The existence of a migraine personality is the subject of some debate. At this time, many physicians believe that there *is* an apparent interaction between personality traits and a biological predisposition for headache pain. The quiz below may help you to find out if some of your personality traits make you more susceptible to migraine.

Before you take the quiz, bear in mind that the word *personality* is being used loosely here. There is no *proven* connection between personality type and headache. The possible migraine personality plays a role only to the extent that stress affects your headaches. In some people, the same stressful feelings or traits may cause ulcer or back pain instead of headache.

The traits and tendencies listed in the quiz can all produce increased levels of stress. If you already have a biological predisposition to headaches, the stresses associated with these personality traits may exacerbate your problem.

1. Do you lead an extremely ordered life?	YES	NO
2. Are you compulsive about anything (cleanliness, punctuality, work, etc.)?	YES	NO
3. Are you rigid or stubborn in your general outlook?	YES	NO
4. Do you dislike change?	YES	NO
5. Do you try to do many things at once?	YES	NO
6. Do you often feel tired?	YES	NO
7. Do you overload easily?	YES	NO
8. Do you suppress feelings of anger?	YES	NO
9. Are you very ambitious or concerned about being successful?	YES	NO
10. Are you a perfectionist?	YES	NO
11. Does your exacting nature make you intolerant of others?	YES	NO

If the great majority of your answers are "yes," you may find yourself more susceptible to migraine attacks than other people.

Since the 1930s, migraine sufferers have been characterized by researchers as obsessive-compulsive. As children, migraine sufferers are reported to be shy, tense, and withdrawn. They are described as simultaneously obedient and defiant, and temper tantrums may result from this frustration. The adult migraine sufferer is characterized as exacting, moralistic, ambitious, and preoccupied with achievement. Conscientious and persistent, often inflexible, this personality type leads an ordered life. *Perfectionist* is a term often used to describe a migraine sufferer. Sexual difficulties may also arise in this personality type.

Throughout most of the 1980s, however, new research has suggested that migraine sufferers may have fairly normal personalities and may be no more neurotic or compulsive than the general population. Some researchers have questioned the previous personality studies and have raised the point that some of the traits often associated with migraine (rigidity, intolerance, anger) may have more to do with the disabling pain the sufferer experiences than with his or her underlying personality.

Furthermore, the samples studied by earlier researchers may not be representative of all migraine sufferers. Only about 50 percent of all migraine sufferers consult physicians. The information collected on the personalities of migraine sufferers, therefore, may be valid only for the type of person who tends to seek medical attention and may have little or no bearing on the rest of migraine sufferers.

Finally, driven "type A" personality traits are related to headaches only to the extent that people react stressfully to them and to the extent that they are already predisposed to headaches. Everyone's appraisal of what constitutes stress is quite different and must be taken into account. For example, two people parachuting out of an airplane may have very different reactions to their potentially stressful situation: One may be terrified, while the other may consider it a sport. Similarly, one achievement-oriented person who overloads his day may remain calm while another with the same activity level may become completely stressed out and possibly suffer a migraine as a result.

THE FORCES BEHIND THE HEADACHE

What causes migraines? The complex physiological process is still somewhat obscure to scientists, but the headaches do seem to be related to vascular changes. A number of factors may directly or indirectly trigger these changes and lead to migraine. These are some of the factors:

Stress and Fatigue

Most headache specialists agree that many migraine patients suffer from stress. Repressed anger and resentment can build up. Stressful situations and changes can bring on attacks in susceptible people. Fatigue and lack of sleep also seem to be culprits—the meticulous, hardworking migraine sufferer may be asking for trouble if she lets herself become too run down. But too much sleep can be as bad as too little: Getting too much sleep can change the body's normally balanced blood sugar levels and trigger headache pain.

Food

Certain foods and beverages are related to migraine attacks in some people, although no one has accurately explained why. Alcohol's link to headache pain is clear: Alcohol is a vasodilator, meaning that blood vessels dilate when alcohol is ingested. This dilation can bring on a vascular headache in migraine sufferers.

The chemical tyramine—found in foods such as aged cheeses, nuts, and yeast—can also cause migraines. The chemical can cause a rise in blood pressure and a pounding headache. A 1970 study found that migraine patients metabolize tyramine differently from normal subjects. This may account for their susceptibility to the effects of tyramine-containing foods. (It should be noted that this sensitivity is not an allergic reaction.)

Fasting can also cause vascular headaches by reducing the sugar content of the blood. Patients with migraines should eat three meals a day and avoid too many carbohydrates. For more on foods to avoid, see pages 74–77.

Hormonal Changes

As many as 60 to 70 percent of female migraine victims report a link between their headache attacks and their menstrual cycles. With some regularity, the headache strikes just before, during, or right at the end of menstruation. The regularity of attacks is the most important indicator of a menstruation-related migraine.

Normally, women's monthly fluctuations in hormonal levels cause no problems; after all, this is what a woman's body was made to do. But in some women, estrogen levels get out of balance. Premenstrual syndrome (PMS) headaches can be triggered by a hormonal imbalance—usually a high level of estrogen in relation to the level of progesterone. Too much estrogen and too little progesterone can cause myriad uncomfortable symptoms, including headache.

Estrogen-containing drugs, such as the pill and certain postmenopausal hormones, may make migraines worse. The use of oral contraceptives is not advised for women suffering from migraine attacks. Check with your gynecologist about this and make sure he or she knows your history of migraines when you discuss contraceptive methods.

PMS, once considered to be "all in a woman's head," is now taken seriously by most doctors. Usually, pregnancy relieves menstruation-related headaches (although in rare cases a woman may experience her first migraine when she is pregnant).

TREATMENT

Don't resign yourself to living with the pain of migraines. Although migraines can be difficult to treat, there is hope. Attacks can be controlled and their frequency lessened (although probably not completely avoided). With persistence, patience, a good doctor, and this book, your attacks should become less frequent and less severe. Treatment must be highly individualized, as the types of migraines and the precipitating factors are different in each case. Depending on the frequency, severity, and type of your attacks, you may want to attempt to control your migraines with nondrug methods first. Some people manage to control their migraines solely through relaxation techniques, diet, and other drug-free methods. If you see a doctor for your migraines, he may suggest that you use preventive methods of treatment to avoid migraines, or "abortive treatment" to help you cope with or stop existing attacks. You may incorporate many nondrug methods of combating migraine into the regimen of drug treatments that your doctor may suggest, should they be necessary.

Nondrug Treatments

Try to avoid the *foods or drinks* that precipitate your headaches (see the chart on pages 75–77).

Changing your normal medications may have a beneficial effect on your headaches. If, for example, birth control pills may be causing your headaches or making them worse, your doctor may suggest discontinuing their use.

Use *relaxation techniques* to help reduce stress and to stop undue muscle tension in the neck, in order to lessen the likelihood of headache pain (see pages 77–80).

Use *stress-reducing techniques* (see pages 80–86) to make your life simpler and happier. A stress-free lifestyle can mean fewer headaches in your life.

Regular exercise (unless your doctor advises against it) can have a positive effect on your circulation, your physical and emotional well-being, and your ability to fight headache pain.

Caffeine is a vasoconstrictive substance and has been known to help some people avoid migraine attacks. It is sometimes included in prescription drugs for treating migraine. Check with your doctor before you try using caffeine to control your headaches; it may or may not be advisable in your case. Excessive caffeine use can *cause* headaches.

For other nondrug methods of treatment, see chapter 8.

Drug Treatments

There are many drugs that can be used to treat or prevent migraines. Which drug you use will depend on your particular case history and your doctor's informed medical opinion. A number of the drugs used for migraine control are listed here for your general information.

The drug *ergotamine tartrate* contains ergot alkaloids and is given to migraine sufferers to stop attacks already in progress. Taken during the prodromal, or aura, phase of the attack, the drug works to constrict the blood vessels, counteracting the dilation that causes the headache pain. It has side effects, however, and precautions must be taken when using it. Large doses can cause nausea, vomiting, diarrhea, and decreased blood supply to the extremities. Ergot alkaloids should not be taken every day. The body may build up a resistance to them, necessitating increased dosages. Finally, the drug may end up actually causing headaches because of a rebound effect associated with overuse. This drug should not be taken by patients with heart disease or a number of other diseases. It should also be avoided if you are pregnant. Be sure to provide your physician with your complete health records and history to ensure a safe treatment plan.

Bellergal combines an ergotamine, a barbiturate, and an antinauseant. It contains very little of the ergotamine and therefore may be used daily without serious risk. However, Bellergal should not be used by anyone who cannot use ergotamine. It also should not be used by anyone with glaucoma because its antinauseant may cause problems.

Midrin is a vasoactive drug; it also combines an analgesic and a sedative for relief from migraine. It consists of acetaminophen, isometheptene mucate, and dichloralphenazone. It may be used by patients unable to use ergots. Even if taken daily, Midrin does not generate a rebound headache.

Methysergide (Sansert), like the ergots, constricts the blood vessels. Hazardous if used over long periods of time, it produces a number of possible side effects, including chest pains, decreased blood flow to the extremities, insomnia, and dizziness. This drug should not be taken during pregnancy or by patients with heart disease, poor circulation, high blood pressure, or lung, liver, or kidney trouble.

Cyproheptadine (Periactin) is an antihistamine that has been proven effective against migraine in many people, including children. It affects the levels of serotonin, the brain chemical that is thought to be at the root of migraines. Cyproheptadine may cause drowsiness or dizziness and should not be taken by people with glaucoma, asthma, or epilepsy, among other conditions.

Propanolol (Inderal), a vasoactive medication, is used to help prevent migraine from occurring. It is the only drug, except for Sansert, approved specifically for headaches. As a beta blocker, propanolol works to lower the effects of stress on the body by lowering blood pressure and preventing dilation of the blood vessels. Like all drugs, propanolol has potential side effects, including asthma attacks, gastrointestinal problems, fatigue, and heart problems. It should not be taken by pregnant women or people with diabetes, asthma, or low blood pressure, among other conditions. In general, however, it has been found to be safe for long-term use.

Clonidine (Catapres) is an alpha blocker. It controls high blood pressure so that vasodilation does not occur. It may cause drowsiness. It should not be used by pregnant women. To discontinue its use, the drug must be phased out slowly rather than stopped suddenly.

Antidepressants such as *amitriptyline* may be taken daily to ward off migraine attacks. Do not think that only depressed people take these drugs. As preventive treatment, amitriptyline does seem to reduce the number of migraine attacks, although this may have to do with the drug's effects on mood or on other migraine-inducing factors. Although most people using this drug do not experience any serious side effects, side effects may include dry mouth, dizziness, tingling, and blurred vision. Its use must be monitored by a doctor, who will do periodic blood tests and physical exams. Amitriptyline may also work well on tension headaches.

Analgesics such as *aspirin, Tylenol,* or *Advil* (ibuprofen) may be tried, but they are rarely very effective since migraine pain stems from dilated blood vessels. Medications that affect the bloodstream seem more effective. Analgesics do help raise the pain threshold, however, and may be helpful for mild migraines.

Drugs for nausea may also be given, if necessary.

DOS AND DON'TS

To take control of your migraine pain, keep the following tips in mind:

- DO keep notes and make charts to help discover the factors that may trigger your headaches.

- DON'T feel resigned to living with migraine pain.

- DO see a doctor for a proper diagnosis of your pain.

- DON'T expect friends and family to automatically understand your struggles. You may have to educate them. Show them this chapter.

- DO try the relaxation techniques and stress reducers listed in chapter 8.

- DON'T aggravate your attacks with alcohol, too little sleep, or too much stress. Try to keep your life on an even keel.

- DO follow your doctor's advice, taking any prescriptions as directed. A treatment plan can't work if you don't follow it.

- DON'T skip meals. When blood sugar levels are low, migraine may be the result. Eat at least three meals a day. Four to six small meals may be even better for you.

- DO avoid foods that can trigger migraine pain, such as aged cheese, nuts, and yeast.

- DON'T take estrogen-containing drugs such as birth control pills, as these might make migraines worse.

- DO seek the help of a gynecologist and/or a headache specialist if you find that your headaches are related to your menstrual cycle.

- DON'T let migraine pain control your life. Take charge now.

FOUR

TENSION HEADACHES

The tension headache is perhaps the most common type of headache. Also known as the muscle contraction headache, it strikes people under emotional stress. Although not usually severe, these headaches can last for days and often begin upon waking in the morning. Unfortunately, these headaches become a chronic, daily pain for some people. Very generally speaking, they are head pains *without* migrainelike symptoms, and they are not related to any underlying diseases. Happily for most sufferers, tension headaches can be treated with fewer medications than other types of headaches.

TIP-OFFS THAT YOU MAY SUFFER FROM TENSION HEADACHES

Check the list of tension headache symptoms below:

- You feel a tight, heavy pressure on your skull, as if you were wearing a hat ten sizes too small.

- Your head aches on both sides, usually on the forehead or the back of the head.

- Your neck and shoulders may hurt as well.

- You are in otherwise normal health.

- The back of your neck knots up during the head-ache. By exploring with your fingers, you may find several tender areas or nodules in the muscles of the head or neck area.

- Warmth or massage applied to your neck and head bring some relief.

- The headache begins without any warning.

- You experience no visual or speech disturbances.

- Neither nausea nor vomiting is present during your attack.

- Your headache often begins during an emotionally trying time period or just after an emotional conflict has ended.

- You may awaken early in the morning with a head-ache, but the headache rarely wakes you up at night. (Only about 10 percent are awakened by pain from a tension headache at night.)

- Your headaches generally began in your adult life (although about 10 percent of sufferers say they had headaches as a child or adolescent).

- The pain of your headache often increases and de-creases throughout the day.

- Your headaches tend to be worse early in the morn-ing and late in the day. They may actually follow a strangely predictable pattern of being more severe between 4 and 8 A.M. and again between 4 and 8 P.M.

Some shared features may blur the distinction be-tween tension headaches and migraines as well as other headache types. Many illnesses are provoked or made worse by emotional tension. Only your doctor can accurately diagnose your pain. This Tip-Off section is not meant to replace such an evaluation.

THE TENSION HEADACHE PERSONALITY

Who is most likely to suffer from tension headaches? Take this quick quiz and find out if *you* are!

1. Do you consider yourself a nervous person?   YES   NO

2. Do your friends and family see you as a
   nervous person?   YES   NO

3. Are you easily angered or frustrated?   YES   NO

4. Do you try to keep your feelings of anger
   and frustration from showing?   YES   NO

5. Are you always in a rush, trying to get
   as much as possible done in one day?   YES   NO

6. Do you often feel depressed or tearful?   YES   NO

7. Does emotional stress bring on your
   headaches?   YES   NO

8. Are you a chronic worrier?   YES   NO

9. Do you often find yourself frowning even
   while you are supposedly relaxing?   YES   NO

10. Do you have any nervous habits such as
    gnashing your teeth or clenching your fists
    or jaw?   YES   NO

11. Do you tend to find fault with everything
    and everyone around you?   YES   NO

12. Is it difficult for you to relax?   YES   NO

13. Do you have trouble relating to other people,
    including close family?   YES   NO

14. Do you have trouble expressing yourself
    openly and honestly?   YES   NO

15. Do you have trouble getting to sleep at night? YES   NO

16. Do you often wake up early, anticipating the
    conflicts of the day?   YES   NO

For years, studies have pointed to anxiety-producing
situations as being at the root of most tension headaches. In a study of one hundred patients experiencing
tension headaches, emotional tension was apparent in
75 percent and depression in 35 percent. Still, other
researchers have raised questions about such findings.
They have pointed out that the patients studied in this
research, being chronic headache sufferers, are poor
test cases: Might not the very fact that they live with
chronic pain cause the emotional tension and depression the researchers see? Either way you look at it,
however, stress and anxiety are strongly linked to the
tension headache.

THE FORCES BEHIND
THE HEADACHE

A tension headache, or muscle contraction headache,
may begin without warning at any time of the day.
The pain is often located in the forehead or at the back
of the head and neck. These headaches have a tendency to occur when a person is under emotional
stress, but the word *tension* in the phrase *tension
headache* refers to muscle tension, not to emotional
tension.

The tension headache was, until recently, blamed
for the contraction of muscles in the scalp, face, or
neck during the headache. Now some researchers believe the contraction may be more a side effect than a
cause. Apparently, stress can cause certain biochemi-
cal changes in the brain, such as decreases in the levels
of the brain chemical serotonin and of endorphins.

Endorphins tend to decrease sensitivity to pain; when endorphin levels are low, a person has a lower pain threshold and may be more susceptible to a headache.

Still, the viselike pain seems linked to the contraction of muscles. Why do muscles contract this way? There is a link between stress and painful muscle contraction, but it can't be scientifically explained. Some have speculated that the muscle contraction is the body's protective response to perceived danger. Much as your heart rate increases when you are frightened, some headache experts believe your neck and head muscles automatically contract during times of stress. When muscles spasm or contract, they can knot up and become tender to the touch. Blood vessels may constrict, reducing the blood supply to the head. Excessive muscle contraction leads to pain that persists long after the muscles relax. Both the muscle contraction and the reduced blood supply play a role in the pain of the tension headache. Other discomforts may worsen the problem, especially if the patient has a mixed tension headache and vascular headache. The blood vessels may periodically dilate and cause a throbbing sensation.

Emotional factors are of great significance in causing tension headaches, but they are not necessarily the *only* agents behind tension headaches. Muscles do not contract only during times of emotional stress. The same pain can be brought on by poor posture or awkward positions of the neck, for example. Driving, watching TV, typing, and reading can all provoke tension headaches because in those activities the neck is often held in a rigid position, with the chin close to the chest. Talking on the telephone by holding the receiver to your ear with a shoulder can also cause excessive muscle contraction and lead to a tension headache.

Certain facial expressions and movements may also lead to headache pain. Prolonged squinting, gum chewing, jaw clenching, and teeth gnashing are all muscle activities that may eventually cause tension headaches.

There is no apparent causal relationship, however, between foods and tension headaches. Nor do we see a connection between hormonal changes and tension headaches, as we do in migraines. Both men and women suffer from tension headaches, although there is a slight predominance of women.

For some people, certain neck diseases or other ailments may be the source of tension headaches, and this should be considered by a doctor. Arthritis of the neck, for example, inflames the joints and may be accompanied by a tension headache. Injuries of the neck, tumors of the spine, and deformities of the vertebrae may also trigger tension headaches.

Sometimes the pain of a migraine headache can cause muscles in the neck and head to contract, thereby adding the discomfort of a tension headache to the agony of a migraine. Some headache experts speculate that this muscle contraction is caused by the body's desire to hold the head immobile during a migraine attack—a protective response that unfortunately causes more pain than it may prevent.

Tension headaches are very rare in children. If a child complains of persistent headaches, help should be sought to look for the underlying cause.

TWO TYPES OF TENSION HEADACHES

Muscle contraction headaches are classified in two types. The *acute* or *episodic* type of tension headache strikes almost everyone at one time or another; very few are immune. Whether brought on by temporary stress, fatigue, or prolonged muscle contraction, the acute tension headache is quite common. It may strike once a month or so and is usually easily dealt with by over-the-counter pain relievers. Only rarely does an episodic sufferer seek the help of a doctor or headache clinic. The pain of an acute tension headache is mild to moderate. The sensation is dull and achey, as if something too tight were squeezing the head. An episodic sufferer may feel the pain in the front of the head, at the sides, on the top of the head, at the back of the head and/or neck, separately, or in any combination.

The *chronic* tension headache is much more disruptive. It can occur daily and often does not respond to over-the-counter pain killers. The chronic sufferer, unlike the episodic sufferer, is likely to seek medical help.

The headache may last for days, weeks, or even months without much relief and may be a sign of depression or anxiety. About 30 percent of chronic tension headache sufferers experience at least one headache a day, and 20 percent have constant pain. The location and severity of the pain are much like what episodic sufferers experience—a tight, viselike feeling in the front, top, or back of the head and sometimes in the sides and neck as well. Sometimes a jabbing pain is also felt.

After the muscle contraction in a chronic headache, the blood vessels may rebound from the reduced blood flow and dilate, causing a throbbing, pounding pain. For the most part, these headaches are not related to underlying health problems. But when a headache is chronic, a doctor will look for physical abnormalities that may be causing the problem, such as TMJ disorders, eye problems, inflammation of the sinuses, physical injuries (such as whiplash or falling on the head), tumors, or neck disorders.

Sometimes physical injuries can damage the occipital nerve, which runs up either side of the neck to behind the ear. When this nerve is damaged, the base of the skull may be tender to the touch and movement of the neck may be restricted. Surgery may be performed to reduce pressure on the nerve.

TREATMENT

Many people with tension headaches do little to avoid or relieve them. Often, episodic sufferers continue their day-to-day activities and wait until the headache ends on its own. Chronic sufferers are less likely to ignore the headaches. When they occur daily, it's hard to overlook the discomfort and pain. Continual headache pain quickly becomes intolerable, and in fact, there is no reason to tolerate it. Help is available for most people.

No one should assume that the mind or the emotions are the sole cause of tension headaches, and a doctor should be consulted to determine whether physical abnormalities or disease is causing the headaches. If an underlying health problem such as TMJ is at the root of the headaches, that problem must be addressed first.

But if no obvious physical abnormality is causing the headaches, they can often be treated without the use of drugs. If certain mental or emotional factors are triggering your headaches, such as tension when you are rushed, you may be able to avoid headaches simply by working on changing your behavior. Biofeedback and stress reduction (described in chapter 8) can significantly curb the frequency of tension headache attacks.

In biofeedback, patients use their thought processes and relaxation techniques to counteract the physical disturbances.

Relaxation exercises and stress reducers can significantly reduce the number of tension headaches in most people. Physical therapy and massage may also be used as preventive measures. Patients can take an active part in these treatments by taking hot showers and massaging their own muscles. But if methods such as these do not work, other treatments must be sought. Most commonly, analgesics (ranging from aspirin to Tylenol to Advil) might then be tried to curb headache pain.

To treat the rarer chronic tension headaches, doctors may prescribe antidepressants and tranquilizers. *Fiorinal* is a brand-name drug that combines a sedative with aspirin; it also contains caffeine. Some drugs, such as *Parafon Forte*, combine the pain relief of acetaminophen with a muscle relaxant. *Darvon* (also a brand name) is a strong pain killer but may lead to addiction and withdrawal problems if overused. *Codeine* is a narcotic pain reliever that is fairly safe but that can also be abused. *Tricyclic antidepressants* have been fairly successful in the treatment of chronic tension headaches. They may work not because of their effect on a person's mood but because of their influence over muscle contractions. It may take a few weeks before the patient recognizes a noticeable difference in headache frequency. *Beta blockers* or *calcium channel blockers* are sometimes prescribed and may be combined with a prescription for an antidepressant. Tranquilizers and muscle relaxants have also been known to work, but their long-term use is discouraged.

Unfortunately, patients sometimes abuse pain relievers and tranquilizers. You must remember that you may cause yourself extra problems if you do so. Prolonged use of these medications can injure the liver, stomach, and kidneys.

DOS AND DON'TS

Here are some dos and don'ts that may help you avoid or control your tension headaches:

- DO maintain good posture.

- DON'T slouch in bed at night peering at TV. Sit up to watch.

- DO look up occasionally from your reading or writing activities so that your neck is not continually held in a chin-to-chest position.

- DON'T prop the telephone between your shoulder and ear.

- DO sleep on a pillow that supports your neck.

- DON'T ignore the basics: good eating and sleeping habits and regular exercise.

- DO practice stress-reducing measures (see pages 80–86).

- DON'T abuse pain killers or tranquilizers in your effort to combat the pain of chronic tension headache.

- DO see a doctor to determine whether physical or emotional factors are triggering your attacks.

- DON'T keep your feelings of anger and frustration in. Express them now, calmly, before you reach a point where you want to explode. See chapter 9.

- DO be receptive to a psychological interview if your doctor thinks one can help you determine emotional factors that may trigger your headaches.

- DON'T let anybody tell you your pain is all in your head.

- DO pursue all avenues to determine possible underlying physical problems before you consider using psychological treatments.

FIVE

CLUSTER HEADACHES

Cluster headaches are relatively rare, affecting far fewer people than the migraine. It is estimated that only about one million people suffer from them, while as many as 16 to 18 million experience migraines.

Medical science has known about cluster headaches for about one hundred years now, but they have been classified under many different and confusing names, including *Raeder's syndrome* and *histamine cephalalgia*. Today we know that cluster headaches are a separate and unique syndrome.

The cluster headache is an extremely painful vascular headache that occurs in groups, or "clusters," of attacks, each usually lasting between fifteen minutes and an hour. Several attacks will occur in one day or daily over several days or weeks. The cluster headache period is usually followed by a long headache-free period. The cluster headache may not return again for as long as three years.

The formidable pain of the headache is almost intolerable and has been described as a boring or piercing sensation, most often located behind one eye. It often causes sufferers to pace about like caged animals and is sometimes bad enough to drive them to bang their heads against walls or even contemplate suicide. It is confined to one side of the head only, in the eye area. Most cluster headache sufferers (about 85 percent) are male, between the ages of twenty and fifty.

TIP-OFFS THAT YOU MAY SUFFER FROM CLUSTER HEADACHES

Check the list of cluster headache symptoms below:

- Your headaches began to occur after your teen years, between the ages of twenty and fifty and most commonly around age thirty.

- Your headache has no preheadache warning phase or sign.

- The intensely painful but short-lived attacks are clustered over a period of days, weeks, or even months. You probably experience between one and three attacks per day, although as many as ten headaches may cluster in a twenty-four-hour period.

- Your headache occurs at the same time every day during the cluster period.

- After the cluster of headaches comes to an end, a headache-free period of up to three years follows.

- You are most likely male. The ratio of male to female sufferers is about six to one. If you are female, your headache has no relationship to your menstrual cycle.

- You are usually the only one in your family to suffer from this type of headache.

- The pain is excruciating.

- The pain is located on one side of your head only.

- The pain is intense around one eye, but some pain may spread to your forehead, temple, or cheek.

- In most attacks, the pain is felt on the same side of the face. (In only about 15 percent of sufferers does it switch sides.)

- The headache pain often wakes you up at night. (According to one source, about 75 percent of attacks take place between nine at night and ten in the morning.)

- During a cluster attack that lasts several days, the headaches occur like clockwork, often at the same time every night.

- Your eye tears.

- Your nose is stuffy but may run at the same time.

- Your face is flushed; there may be sweat on your forehead.

- The eyelid on the affected side of your head droops and may look puffy.

- Your eye is often bloodshot.

- The pupil temporarily shrinks in size, and your vision may be blurred.

- Your heart rate speeds up.

- There is sometimes seasonal regularity to the appearance of your headaches. Your headaches may be more prevalent in spring and fall.

- Drinking alcohol during your headache period can trigger the pain.

To further highlight the properties of the cluster headache, the chart below compares them with migraines. This should help you to clearly understand the differences between these two types of vascular headache. The cluster headache is clinically different from a migraine and should not be confused with any other headache type.

Feature	Cluster Headache	Migraine Headache
Location in head	Always unilateral (one-sided)	Unilateral or bilateral
Age of sufferer at onset	20 to 50 years	10 to 40 years
Male/female incidence	90% male	65% to 70% female
Occurrence of attacks	Daily, for several weeks or months	Intermittent, 2 to 8 times per month
Duration of pain	10 minutes to 3 hours	4 to 48 hours
Prodromes (pre-headache warning signs)	None	25% to 30% of cases
Nausea and vomiting	2% to 5% of cases	85% of cases
Blurring of vision	Infrequent	Frequent
Eye tearing	Frequent	Infrequent
Nasal congestion	Frequent	Uncommon
Family history of vascular headaches	7% of cases	90% of cases

Adapted from a chart compiled by Dr. Seymour Diamond, director of the Diamond Headache Clinic in Chicago.

TRAITS OF THE
CLUSTER HEADACHE SUFFERER

As doctors researched cluster headaches, they found unusual similarities among their patients who suffered from them, peculiar findings whose significance medical science is still unable to explain. A 1972 study by a researcher named Graham confirmed that most of the sufferers are big, muscular men. The men are taller than average. They often have a rugged appearance that has been described as lionlike. They commonly have a square jaw and a cleft chin. Their skin is coarse, with texture like that of an orange peel. Their foreheads are often deeply furrowed. Even their eye color is similar: Most men with cluster headaches have light-colored eyes, of blue or green.

Perhaps the most startling similarity is that as many as 94 percent of cluster headache sufferers smoke cigarettes. Furthermore, they smoke heavily, puffing about thirty-two cigarettes a day. Most are two- to three-pack-a-day smokers. Often, they began to smoke in the teen years. They also tend to be heavy drinkers.

So far, these similarities are strictly observations. No one knows why people with these physical characteristics and habits are more susceptible to cluster headaches. Connections between the similarities and the headaches remain basically unclear, but doctors sometimes use the pattern to help them diagnose cluster headache sufferers. It is also not understood why drinking alcohol triggers pain during a cluster headache period but has no apparent effect during headache-free periods.

THE FORCES BEHIND
THE HEADACHE

The cluster headache is a cyclical disorder. All the current evidence indicates that this syndrome stems from problems in a person's biological clock. The biological clock theory emerged, in part, because of the cyclical nature of the headaches and the fact that they often occur at the same time of day during the cycle.

The body's biological clock regulates enzyme activities, body temperature, and hormone secretions as well as other physiological behavior. In cluster headache victims, the body seems to have some difficulty controlling these natural rhythms. The hypothalamus, which controls sleep and wakefulness, may be at the root of this conundrum. The hypothalamus may send a central-nervous-system discharge into the bloodstream; this causes the blood vessels to dilate. But the dilation of the blood vessels is thought to be the result, not the cause, of the trouble. Serotonin levels may be another factor; this brain chemical, along with histamine, regulates the biological clock and is connected anatomically to the eye.

Histamine levels may also be involved. Histamine is a vasoactive substance found primarily in the hypothalamus; it dilates the blood vessels. Researchers have discovered that injecting a small amount of histamine into a cluster headache patient triggers a headache. This fact is cited as evidence of a link between histamine and headache.

Many cluster headache patients say that they are awakened at night by their headaches. In about half of the cases, researchers estimate, this awakening occurs during REM, or rapid eye movement, sleep. No one knows why this is so.

Alcohol, a vasodilator, can precipitate the headaches during a cluster cycle. Patients are warned against drinking during a cluster headache period.

TWO TYPES OF CLUSTER HEADACHES

Although most sufferers experience cluster headaches only occasionally, with long periods of respite between bouts, some develop a chronic problem. Chronic cluster headaches plague the victim continually and grant no headache-free period. It is the severity and relentlessness of this chronic pain that causes people to consider suicide. Happily, only about 10 percent of cluster headache victims develop a chronic problem. Their problem, however, is very difficult to treat and surgery may be suggested.

TREATMENT

Cluster headaches can be hard to treat because they come on rapidly and without warning. Furthermore, the pain often wakes the victim from sleep, which makes it hard to take the measures needed to abort the attack.

Fortunately, many sufferers can be treated without drugs. Oxygen inhalation by face mask is the initial treatment of choice, and it works in about 70 to 80 percent of cases. For this treatment to be effective, the sufferer must inhale five to eight liters of 100 percent oxygen per minute for ten to fifteen minutes. Oxygen has a vasoconstrictive effect on neurotransmitters, and it may short-circuit the painful dilation of the blood vessels. Oxygen also stimulates the production of serotonin in the central nervous system, which may help as well. Using this treatment obviously necessitates that an oxygen tank be on the premises when you get an attack. Often this is not possible or convenient.

Vigorous physical exercise at the earliest sign of a cluster headache has also been reported to be effective in aborting an attack. Applying pressure to the temporal artery has been reported to relieve pain temporarily in about 40 percent of cases but to worsen the pain in another 40 percent of cases. During a cluster attack, avoiding drinking alcohol (which is known to dilate blood vessels) can decrease the number of headaches. Foods that contain vasoactive ingredients should also be avoided.

If these nondrug methods prove unsatisfactory, drugs are also available for use in preventing or aborting the cluster headache syndrome. Some of the drugs used to abort cluster headaches during the course of an attack are *somatostatin, ergotamine, cocaine hydrochloride*, and *lidocaine*. Lidocaine is administered as a nose drop during an attack and is effective in four out of five patients. It is often preferable, however, to use drugs to prevent attacks rather than to abort one already in progress. Medications that control vascular activity work best. Preventive drugs that may be used include *methysergide (Sansert), cyproheptadine, verapamil, corticosteroids, prednisone,* and *triamcinolone*. Methysergide is about 70 percent effective for occasional cluster headache sufferers but does not work well for chronic sufferers. Steroids are effective but are given only for short periods of time; they help break the cycle of headaches because of their effect on neurotransmitters. *Lithium carbonate* may be an effective treatment for chronic cluster headaches.

Histamine desensitization has also been tried as a therapy. In histamine desensitization, small doses of histamine are given intravenously to build up resistance to its effects. But this treatment's effectiveness is open to question, and it has been for the most part abandoned. Scientists are also questioning whether its occasional effectiveness was not simply a placebo effect. Today it is used only under select conditions and is tried only in chronic cases.

In serious cases of chronic suffering from cluster headaches, a new surgery is available called *radio frequency trigeminal rhizotomy*. The surgery works to kill pain sensors in the affected area. A needle is placed in the trigeminal nerve of the brain, and microwavelike radio frequency waves are applied. The waves kill pain-carrying fibers of the nerve, which remain numb to pain. This is a very precise operation and must be performed by a neurosurgeon. Seventy percent of patients having this operation find it extremely successful. The surgery is rarely recommended and is reserved only for chronic sufferers, as it causes numbness of the facial muscles.

OTHER HEADACHES

There are several other types and varieties of headaches from which you may be suffering.

FOOD-RELATED HEADACHES

A number of common foods seem to trigger headaches in some people, including some hard cheeses, citrus fruits, alcohol, Chinese food, and chocolate, among others. Headache-provoking foods all contain substances known as amines (such as tyramine and phenylethylamine), which can trigger headaches. Food additives that seem to precipitate headaches include sodium chloride, monosodium glutamate (MSG), sodium nitrite, and aspartame. In the future, we may discover other chemicals that are responsible for bringing on headache pain.

Hot Dog Headache

Some people experience headache pain following a meal of hot dogs or other processed meats. These meats contain nitrites, a preservative that can cause dilation of the blood vessels. Foods that are likely to contain nitrites include hot dogs, canned meats, salami, bologna, sausage, bacon, pepperoni, and smoked fish. Check the labels on meat products to find out whether they contain nitrites.

Chinese Restaurant Headache

The chemical monosodium glutamate (MSG) is commonly used in Chinese cooking as a flavor enhancer. It is also found in many canned foods, meat tenderizers, and seasoned salts. Unfortunately, about 10 to 30 percent of people who eat MSG will get a headache. This reaction usually takes the form of a sequence of symptoms, beginning with a burning sensation that moves over the chest, neck, and shoulders. Next, the chest becomes tight. Then the head and face experience the same tightness and pressure.

It is not clear why MSG has this effect on some individuals; it seems to have no impact on arterial walls. To avoid the headache, when you go to a Chinese restaurant, ask that your food be prepared without MSG—most restaurants will accommodate you. Some studies have found that if a person eats something else before eating a Chinese meal, MSG absorption is slowed and may not result in a headache. One study found that drinking alcohol at the same time as eating food with MSG may make a headache more likely to occur. Soy sauce also causes headaches in some people. Keep these points in mind to avoid the Chinese restaurant headache.

Vitamin A Headache

Vitamin A overdoses can cause severe headaches, often accompanied by abdominal pain, nausea, and dizziness. The headache syndrome disappears once vitamin A is no longer being taken. Beware—almost any vitamin in large doses is dangerous, so avoid megadoses. Let your doctor know how many vitamins you take each day.

Ice Cream Headache

As many people know, eating ice cream or drinking a frosty drink can cause a sudden and unexpected headache. This headache is more likely to occur if the weather is very hot or if the person is overheated. The pain—which feels as if it comes from deep within the head—can hit as quickly as twenty-five to sixty seconds after ingesting the cold substance.

The ice cream hits the warm roof of the mouth and apparently causes a vascular reaction that in turn causes the pain. Happily, the head pain lasts only a minute or so. About one-third of the general population experiences ice cream headaches occasionally, but as many as 90 percent of people susceptible to migraine have this reaction to excessively cold foods and drinks. Some people find the headaches annoying enough that they eliminate cold foods from their diets altogether. Others simply exercise a little caution by stirring ice cream into a slightly warmer, soupier form before eating it.

Hangover Headache

The hangover headache is caused by alcohol. (It is not the same as a migraine or cluster headache that may be *triggered* by alcohol.) Only some people are susceptible to this effect. Alcohol may cause a headache about thirty minutes after consumption in some, or—more commonly—it may cause a hangover headache many hours later, usually the morning after. A person need not drink a lot of alcohol to experience a hangover. Alcohol can cause headaches because it leads to dilation of the blood vessels. There is some speculation that the hangover headache is actually a withdrawal symptom. The headache caused by a hangover is usually accompanied by nausea, lightheadedness, fatigue, pallor, dehydration, and a general feeling of malaise. The hangover headache usually strikes both sides of the head with a throbbing pain. The headache often feels worse when the head is moved. Within five to ten hours, the sufferer usually feels better.

Apparently, some alcoholic drinks are more likely to cause hangover headaches than others. Beer, red wine, and sherry, for example, may be more likely than vodka because they contain more amines. If you plan to drink, you may lessen the likelihood of getting a hangover by eating something beforehand. Fruits and honey are apparently the best foods to eat, as their fructose helps the body to burn off the alcohol faster.

To treat a hangover, try drinking a caffeinated drink like coffee, which constricts the dilated blood vessels and lessens head pain. Ice packs on the head are also effective. Contrary to popular belief, taking another drink does not help and only makes the hangover worse. Not surprisingly, very few studies have been done on this extremely common problem. Perhaps we consider a headache to be a fair price to pay for a night of revelry.

OTHER HEADACHES

Cough Headache

Some people experience head pain when they cough, sneeze, lift, bend, or stoop. At one time, doctors thought this was almost always indicative of a serious underlying health problem. Today, however, the majority of cases are considered to be basically benign. Magnetic resonance imaging (MRI) of the head is usually done just to be sure because in rare cases a serious problem such as a brain tumor is the cause of the cough headache. About 10 percent of cough headache patients discover an underlying disease at the root of their pain. Cough headaches reach their peak right away and disappear within a few minutes.

Exertion Headache

A number of people experience headaches after doing strenuous activity. Exertion headaches, sometimes also called effort migraines, begin suddenly after prolonged physical activity, such as running. The effort migraine is more likely to last hours than minutes. Treatment may involve using an antimigraine medication. *Indomethacin* (Indocin) has been cited as being particularly helpful.

Fever Headache

The headache caused by fever is considered a toxic vascular headache. The fever dilates blood vessels in the head, causing a painful throbbing sensation. When the fever is reduced, the head pain is too.

"Not Tonight, Dear" Headache

Some headaches seem to be associated with sexual activity. They occur just before or during orgasm and are a sudden, throbbing pain in the back part of the head. Luckily, these headaches occur only infrequently in sufferers and are rarely a regular result of sex. It is possible that sexual activity is simply a trigger for a cough headache. Men are much more likely to suffer from them than are women. These headaches also tend to strike migraine sufferers.

The headache may last from a few minutes to hours. Some speculate that at least some of these headaches are caused by muscle contraction and tension in the head and neck during sex. The more painful headaches that occur at orgasm may be due to hypertension. This type of headache is rarely the result of a serious problem, but in some instances an aneurysm is responsible for the pain. This possibility must be checked out by a doctor before an accurate diagnosis or treatment can be given.

Sunshine Headache

Sitting in the sun causes throbbing headaches in some people. This headache is not to be confused with the migraine, which is triggered by glare. In light of this and more serious dangers associated with sun exposure, including skin cancer, people are advised to exercise caution and stay out of the sun. Wearing a hat when outdoors helps decrease sun exposure and lessen the likelihood of a sunshine headache. Wearing high-quality sunglasses that cut glare and filter out the sun's rays provides added protection outdoors.

Constipation Headache

People who become constipated often experience a headache at the same time. The headache that accompanies constipation is dull and throbbing. No one knows quite why they occur, although some speculate that toxic substances from the stool become absorbed into the bloodstream; others suggest that emotional upset and depression may cause the headaches. (People who are depressed are also more likely to suffer from constipation.)

Constipation has become a common problem, with the average American diet low in fiber and high in refined foods. Constipation and the associated headaches may be avoided by eating whole grains, legumes, fruits, and vegetables—all high-fiber foods. Refined and processed foods, such as white sugar, white rice, and white bread, should be avoided.

PMS Headache

For many women, the days right before their periods are marred by uncomfortable feelings of bloating, back pain, depression, irritability, and headache. Headache symptoms that surface about a week before menstruation and then dissipate by the end of the period may be caused by premenstrual syndrome, or PMS. PMS is a series of symptoms (over 150 have been identified) that begin around the time of ovulation and disappear during the period or just after it. Only a physician can accurately diagnose PMS, but you should consider yourself a sufferer if the onset of and relief from your discomforts is cyclically regular.

PMS is triggered by hormonal imbalances. At ovulation, estrogen and progesterone levels are on the rise. Estrogen is the female hormone that stimulates the ovaries to produce a new egg each month; the hormone progesterone thickens the lining of the uterus in anticipation of pregnancy. If there is no pregnancy, the progesterone level falls, and menstruation begins. PMS occurs when this normal equilibrium gets off balance and there is too much estrogen and not enough progesterone in the body (see pages 30–31.)

Treatments that are being tried for PMS, with mixed results, include stress management, diet, exercise, and sometimes antidepressants. If water retention is a problem, some women are given diuretics and told to avoid salty foods and to restrict fluid intake. Nutritional and vitamin therapy (calcium, magnesium, vitamin B_6) works for some. Other nondrug treatments include yoga, rest, and a caffeine-free diet. One of the newest treatments for PMS is gamma linoleic acid, or oil of evening primrose, taken in capsule form. Responses to treatment are highly individualized.

You may want to see both a gynecologist who specializes in PMS and a headache specialist. PMS treatment centers (physician-directed, all-inclusive centers with psychiatrists, nutritionists, gynecologists, and nurses) are springing up around the country. (The centers usually charge a flat rate for a three-to-six-month treatment program or may charge on a per visit basis.)

Headaches in Children

Children get headaches too. A child's headaches, like an adult's, may be caused by any number of factors including fatigue, fever, ear infections, eating certain foods, hunger, or overexcitement. The child should see a doctor to determine the cause. Usually, treatment is confined to nutritional guidelines and acetaminophen for pain relief.

SEVEN

HEADACHES WITH ORGANIC CAUSES

Almost everyone who suffers from headaches at one time or another worries about the possibility of brain tumor or other serious illness. Happily, these are rarely the cause. Only 2 percent of headaches brought to doctors' attention are caused by such diseases.

BRAIN TUMOR

A brain tumor is not likely to be the cause of your headache. Only an estimated 0.1 to 0.5 percent of those who seek help for a headache actually have a tumor. A patient with a tumor experiences more symptoms than just headache, including dizziness, nausea, blurred vision, seizures, paralysis, and personality changes. Nausea and vomiting may accompany it, but this occurs in migraine as well. The pain of a headache need not be severe to indicate tumor, but it may worsen with exertion. If you are experiencing neurological symptoms such as numbness or seizures along with your headaches, you will certainly want your doctor to check out the possibility of a tumor. Usually, your doctor's examination will rule out the possibility of tumor right away, but more tests may be required, such as a CAT (computerized axial tomography) scan, magnetic resonance imaging, or a skull X ray.

Treatment depends on the type of tumor present.

TEMPORAL ARTERITIS

The temporal arteritis headache is caused by inflamed arteries in the head and neck. It affects mostly people in their fifties or older. The pain is deep and throbbing, with a burning or sometimes jabbing sensation. Facial swelling and scalp tenderness may accompany the headache. You may also experience pain in chewing, a stiff neck, fatigue, or loss of weight. Temporal arteritis is a potentially serious problem that may lead to stroke or blindness and requires prompt attention. If you are in the fifty-plus age group and have only recently begun to have headaches, your doctor will probably test you for this disease with a blood test known as a sedimentation rate. If the test results indicate that it is necessary, a temporal artery biopsy may be performed.

The condition often responds to small doses of steroids (cortisone compounds). If the headaches improve and the sedimentation rate declines with this treatment, the drug is gradually discontinued. To make sure the disease has been checked, sedimentation rate tests are performed even after the patient is off the medication.

STROKE

Very rarely, a headache is a warning of bleeding into or around the brain. The bleeding may extend into the brain itself, possibly mixing with the cerebrospinal fluid. The bleeding may be due to a burst aneurysm or blood vessel. The headaches may be accompanied by a decrease in consciousness, and there may also be stiff neck or neck pain. Depending on where the blood travels, there may also be back and leg pain.

HYPERTENSION

Unusually high blood pressure can cause headaches. More important than treating the headaches is treating the high blood pressure itself. Unfortunately, some of the drugs used to control high blood pressure can themselves cause headaches. If you are on medication for high blood pressure and are experiencing headaches, consult your doctor.

MENINGITIS

Meningitis is an inflammation of the brain's tissue covering. Headache is just one of the many symptoms of meningitis. High fever, a flulike condition, fatigue, vomiting, a stiff neck, and sensitivity to light are also symptoms. There are two types of meningitis—viral and bacterial. Viral meningitis is not as serious, and the patient recovers fairly quickly. Bacterial meningitis (or spinal meningitis) is another matter entirely—it is a serious and often life-threatening infection that needs immediate medical attention and treatment with antibiotics.

SINUSITIS

Sinusitis is an infection that causes inflammation of sinus tissues, swelling of the blood vessels, and blockage of mucus flow. Pus forms within the sinus cavities and cannot drain. People with sinusitis are likely to also have a fever.

A sinusitis headache often accompanies the blocked sinus passages. The pain is usually felt just above and below the eyes, where the sinuses are located.

Although many people think they suffer from sinus headaches, only about one in fifty people who seek help for them actually has sinusitis. Doctors blame this confusion on the abundance of aspirin advertisements that describe sinus headache pain. In fact, many headache conditions, including migraine, can cause these same sinus-related symptoms. Sinusitis is diagnosed when an X ray of the sinuses shows blockage. If tests indicate that you do have sinusitis, you will be referred to an ear, nose, and throat doctor, or otorhinolaryngologist. Treatment may include antibiotics for the infections, decongestants, and antihistamines. The specialist may have to drain your sinuses mechanically or, in some cases, perform surgery.

TEMPOROMANDIBULAR
JOINT DISORDER (TMJ)

The increasingly talked-about disease TMJ involves muscle tension in the jaw joint. Headache is the most common symptom of TMJ. The pain is usually felt at the base of the head, at the back of the neck, or behind the ear. TMJ, most often brought about by an improperly aligned bite or by dental habits such as nighttime teeth grinding, should be treated by a dentist with expertise in the field. Because some people believe TMJ is overdiagnosed, it is advisable to stay in touch with a general doctor or headache specialist as well; it may be that your head pain is *not* TMJ-related after all. Some of the treatments for TMJ include exercise of the joint, bite plates, massage, heat therapy, sedatives, and muscle relaxants. Rarely, surgery is suggested.

TIC DOULOUREUX
(TRIGEMINAL NEURALGIA)

Tic douloureux affects the nerves of the face and can be very painful. Both men and women suffer, usually over the age of fifty. Sufferers experience recurring jabs or flashes of intense pain on one side of the face. The pain can be triggered by touch, and patients may avoid brushing their teeth, shaving, applying makeup, and so on to escape the pain. The cause of the condition is uncertain, except that a painful message is being sent by the trigeminal nerves. Treatment depends on the severity of the condition and its response to medication. An anticonvulsant may be recommended, and sometimes surgery is suggested on the trigeminal nerve, which may cause facial numbness.

EYESTRAIN AND
EYE DISEASE

The pain of some headaches is located in the eyes, not the head. A thorough eye exam is almost always a good diagnostic tool, as pain from eye disease and even eyestrain can cause headache. On the other hand, pain from other areas of the head can also cause pain in the eye area.

Eyestrain can be a cause of headaches. In these cases, habits such as reading in inadequate light or not wearing glasses may be at the root of the pain. Eyestrain can also occur if you need glasses but don't have a prescription for them yet. If you think this is your problem, see an eye specialist to have your sight tested and glasses prescribed if necessary. Fluorescent lighting, with its imperceptible flickering, triggers eyestrain headaches in some people. Glaring light or bright sunlight can also bring on headache pain. If the pain is being caused by eyestrain, there is usually a noticeable improvement after eyes are rested, glasses are used, or a new prescription is filled.

Glaucoma is another, more serious cause of headaches. Glaucoma causes pressure within the eye, and vision often becomes foggy. It can eventually cause blindness if left untreated. It does not strike the elderly alone; young people suffer from glaucoma as well.

If glaucoma is suspected, a simple test is given to measure the amount of pressure within the eye. Many doctors now recommend that the glaucoma test be administered annually to all adults, whether or not glaucoma is suspected. Treatments include medication and surgery. Some headache medications can make certain types of glaucoma worse, and for this and other reasons, the glaucoma test is very important. These drugs include antihistamines, antinauseants, some tranquilizers, some laxatives, antidepressants, and others. Check with your doctor about this if you are affected.

HYPOGLYCEMIA

Hypoglycemia is not a disease but a condition, of low blood sugar. One symptom may be headache pain. Hypoglycemia can be a sign of many underlying health problems, including pancreatic tumors and liver disease; it is sometimes an early sign of diabetes. Although some think it is a common problem, low blood sugar is in reality fairly rare.

Low blood sugar is occasionally the cause of headache pain. Its symptoms include, besides head pain, light-headedness, dizziness, sweating, and sometimes even loss of consciousness. Many physicians believe that the media have exaggerated the prevalence of hypoglycemia, causing people to incorrectly believe that they have hypoglycemia. The test for hypoglycemia is a five-hour oral glucose test, which measures blood sugar levels.

People who experience headaches as a result of missed meals are not necessarily hypoglycemic. Migraine sufferers, for example, often get headaches if they go without food. This does not mean that they have hypoglycemia. Headaches that result from skipped meals or long stretches without eating can be avoided by eating four to six small meals during the day. A high-protein snack before bedtime may help improve the morning headaches that can come about after an overnight with no food.

Now that you are familiar with the many and varied types of headaches, you'll want to know more about the types of treatments available. It's time to stop suffering passively. With the help of the next chapter, you may be able to avoid your headaches without using drugs.

EIGHT

NONDRUG METHODS OF PAIN RELIEF

Right now, your headaches may seem like an insurmountable force controlling your life. But there *are* ways to take charge and help yourself, many ways to control and combat headaches, and they needn't involve doctors and drugs. Both doctors and headache sufferers have invented and used various nondrug methods of headache relief. These "home remedies" have had varying rates of success, and some may work for you.

Both you and your doctor probably would like to avoid drug treatment for your headaches unless it becomes necessary. You will certainly be far better off if drug-free methods work for you. Drug dependence can become a very real and serious problem for headache sufferers who have to use them for pain relief. Many of the pain-killing drugs available for alleviating headaches—including over-the-counter medications—require increasingly large doses as the patient develops a tolerance for them. Worse, when the drug is discontinued, unpleasant withdrawal symptoms may result.

Aspirin is probably the most overused drug. Although it is seemingly harmless, overuse may lead to kidney failure. Prescription drugs may become addictive, especially those that combine analgesics with tranquilizers. This is not to say that all drugs should be uniformly refused; many headache sufferers need medication to prevent or control headaches. The warning is simply against continual and habitual use of a drug.

For this and other reasons, it is prudent to try drug-free methods before turning to drugs. Sufferers have found relief using all of the following nondrug methods: exercise, changes in sleep habits, acupuncture/acupressure, biofeedback, ice packs, heating pads, relaxation techniques, massage, sex, hypnosis, meditation, food avoidance, low-sugar/high-protein diets with frequent small meals, chiropractic adjustments, handwarming, and even herbal remedies. Hopefully, one will work for you.

FOOD PLAYS AN IMPORTANT ROLE IN HEADACHE CONTROL

Many people have found that the food they eat or don't eat affects the frequency and severity of their headaches. A number of sufferers, for example, have found that eliminating tyramine from their diet can help a great deal—tyramine being a vasoactive substance that is contained in a variety of foods. The chart gives general information about foods that seem to trigger headaches in some patients. It indicates which foods to avoid and suggests foods to try in their place. If it is not possible for you to avoid these foods, you might try limiting your intake. Be sure to check with your doctor before beginning any dietary plan. Only your doctor can determine the safety of this plan for you.

Foods to Avoid	*Foods to Try Instead*
cheddar cheese	American cheese
gruyere	Velveeta or other processed cheese
brie	ricotta
other ripened cheeses	cottage cheese
	cream cheese
yogurt	limit to ½ cup yogurt
sour cream	imitation sour cream
buttermilk	
chocolate milk	
bologna	fresh meats
salami	
pepperoni	
hot dogs	
pork	
other smoked or processed meats	
chicken livers	
pickled herring	
avocados	restrict to ½ banana per day,
bananas	½ grapefruit, ½ cup orange
papayas	juice
grapefruit	
oranges	
other citrus fruits, drinks	

Foods to Avoid	Foods to Try Instead
pinto beans	
lima beans	
navy beans	
garbanzo beans	
pea pods	
nuts	
peanut butter	
sunflower seeds	
sesame seeds	
pumpkin seeds	
raisins	
onions	
sauerkraut	
yeast	
sourdough bread	commercial breads
raised doughnuts	
homemade fresh bread	
beer	Although all alcohol should
sherry	be avoided, the least
red wine*	offensive is vodka.
bourbon	nonalcoholic wines and beers
other alcoholic drinks	

*According to one study, white wine does not bring on migraine attacks the way red wine can.
NOTE: This chart was prepared with assistance from the Diamond Headache Clinic.

Foods to Avoid	*Foods to Try Instead*
MSG (found in many canned foods as well as in most Chinese food)	request "no MSG" when ordering Chinese food
soy sauce	
vinegar	
pickled foods	
chocolate	
coffee	decaffeinated coffee,
tea	herbal teas,
other caffeinated drinks	decaffeinated soda, noncaffeinated beverages

RELAXATION CAN WORK WONDERS

Tension can cause or worsen headaches because our bodies react physically to stress. During times of stress, blood vessels and muscles may contract, causing pain. This is actually a throwback to Neanderthal days, when threats of danger were quite real and a physical reaction, such as fleeing or fighting, was necessary for survival. The threatened caveman's heart would speed up, his blood pressure would rise, and his pupils would dilate, all in preparation for action. Today, even though many of the dangers of Neanderthal times are gone, our physical response to tense situations remains about the same.

This physical reaction to stress is known as a *sympathetic response*. Relaxation methods can be used to reverse it. Some headaches sufferers have been able to get remarkable relief in this way. You can learn to increase what is known as your *parasympathetic response*, which opens up the flow of blood and calms you, by using relaxation techniques.

A parasympathetic response that comes too late and too strong, however, may be at the root of migraine pain. (It is theorized that after the initial vasoconstriction, which may cause the visual disturbances prior to the migraine, the parasympathetic response kicks in, ballooning the arteries and causing the pounding pain we associate with migraine.) The trick is in *early* parasympathetic intervention.

Relaxation can be harder for some people to achieve than it sounds. Fortunately, you train yourself to unwind using exercises. With a little training and forethought, you should be able to leave your tension behind. Some of the following exercises may get you to relax.

The Breath of Fresh Air

Inhale deeply through your nose as you count to eight. Then pucker your lips and exhale slowly to the count of sixteen—longer if you can. Concentrate on the sound of your breath, and try to imagine the tension dissolving as you blow out. Repeat ten times.

The Swinging Door

Sit quietly and comfortably. Visualize a pair of swinging doors. Inhale as you imagine the doors swinging in. Exhale as the doors swing out. Continue breathing in time to the swinging doors. As you watch the doors, if any other thoughts come into your mind, let them come in and go right out again. Allow yourself to sag. Relax. The swinging doors become hypnotic, keeping your breathing regular.

The Rag Doll

Sit or lie down. Start at the tippy-top of your head and say to yourself, *Relax your forehead, relax your jaw, relax your mouth, relax your neck,* and so on. Concentrate on relaxing each part of your body, one at a time. Soon you will be as limp as a rag doll.

Opposites Attract

This is an exercise of tension and relaxation. Often we aren't aware of the muscle tension in our bodies. This exercise makes you aware of the tension and gives you a sense of what a relaxed state should feel like.

Choose a part of your body, such as your jaw. Clench your jaw, grit your teeth, and make the muscles tense. Then relax the same muscles. Feel the difference. Pick another part of your body, such as an arm. Tighten it, then let it go. Again, note the difference.

A Real Glass Act

Sit still, and concentrate on your breathing. Imagine your face becoming as smooth as glass, with not a wrinkle or a crack. Imagine your face as a glassy lake, totally undisturbed.

The Five-Minute Vacation

Imagine that you are on a beach. Watch the surf roll up and back, up and back. Concentrate on your quiet beach for at least five minutes, relaxing this way.

The Meltdown

Sit in a chair. Close your eyes, and breathe slowly. Place your hand on your belly and feel it rise and fall with each breath. As you inhale, your hand is pushed up. As you exhale, your hand sinks back down. You are now breathing from your diaphragm instead of from your chest.

The Secret Password

Use the diaphragm-breathing technique from "The Meltdown." As you exhale, silently repeat one word over and over, such as *calm, relax, peace, hush, harmony, tranquillity,* or *gentle.*

STRESS REDUCERS

Stress is a universal response, and sometimes it is unavoidable. Unfortunately, high stress levels trigger headaches in many people.

Much depends on a person's reaction to stress. A demanding boss may upset some people, but the same boss may be a challenge to others. *Stress* is not necessarily a dirty word, and a little bit can provide positive stimulation. But when it begins to interfere with your enjoyment of life, you need to rethink the way you respond to things. A less stressful life can significantly improve your headache situation. The following stress-reducing tips, provided with the help of the National Headache Foundation, can help you put your life on an even keel and may reduce the number of headache episodes you normally experience. Reduce your anxiety and frustration by following these tips, but remember that not all of them apply to you. Figure out what causes the most stress in your life, and apply the appropriate stress reducer to your circumstances.

- Get up fifteen minutes earlier than usual each morning. Being less rushed, you will avoid the stress of early morning hassles and mishaps. You might even want to prepare for the morning the night before. Set the breakfast table, lay out the clothes you plan to wear, place your work papers back in your briefcase, and the like. An orderly morning lessens the day's aggravations.

- Don't rely on your memory. Instead, keep a calendar on which you write down appointment times, when to pick up the laundry, when library books are due, and so on. That way you won't constantly have that anxious feeling that there's something you *should* be doing but can't remember what it is.

- Make a duplicate of your house key and hide it somewhere in your yard. Carry a duplicate car key in your wallet. You'll never have to worry about being locked out of the house or the car again.

- Practice preventive maintenance so that your car, appliances, and home will be less likely to break down or fall apart at the "worst possible moment." As an ounce of prevention, always keep the kitchen stocked with emergency staples (enough at least for a tuna casserole or spaghetti and sauce) so you'll never be *totally* out of food for dinner.

- Be prepared for lines and unavoidable waits. Carry a paperback or magazine with you for reading pleasure so you can make the time pass more agreeably—without grinding your teeth!

- Procrastination is stressful. Whatever you want to put off for tomorrow, do today. Plan ahead! Don't let the gas tank drop below one-quarter full. Don't wait until you're down to your last token or last stamp to buy more.

- Don't put up with something that doesn't work right. If your alarm clock, windshield wipers, toaster oven—whatever—is a constant aggravation, get it fixed or get a new one!

- Don't run late. Give yourself fifteen minutes of extra time to get to appointments, trains, and planes. Plan to arrive at an airport one hour before your domestic flight leaves.

- Make contingency plans, "just in case." For example, tell your partner, "If for some reason either one of us is delayed, here's what we'll do." Or, "If we get split up while shopping, here's where we'll meet."

- Relax your standards. Contrary to popular belief, not all things worth doing are worth doing well. Maybe your checkbook needn't be balanced to the last penny. Be a little more flexible. Perfection is not always attainable, and even when it is, it is not always valuable. The world will not end if the dishes don't get washed tonight, if the bed doesn't get made this morning, or if the lawn doesn't get mowed this weekend.

- Count your blessings! For every single thing that went wrong today, probably ten or fifty or more things went right! The baby-sitter came on time, you remembered your umbrella, you caught the early train. Think of these things. Remembering the good things can reduce your aggravation when you're up against the one thing that *didn't* go your way.

- Get it right the first time. Repeat back directions, and ask questions about a task assigned to you. If you do something right the first time through, you'll save yourself hours of time and perhaps a headache as well!

- Learn to say no. Say no to an extra project, a speech you don't really want to give, a social engagement you don't have time for. This may take some practice and restraint on your part, especially if you're used to doing it all. But a little time off is necessary to reduce stress.

- Unplug your phone. This is harder to do than it sounds. But if you want to have an uninterrupted sleep, bath, or moment of silence, disconnect yourself from the outside world. The possibility that a terrible emergency will occur in the next hour is almost nil. More likely, a talkative insurance salesman or pesky neighbor will try to call you.

- Make friends with nonworriers. Nothing can get you into the habit of worrying faster than fretting with other chronic worrywarts.

- While you are working, get up and stretch periodically. Don't sit scrunched in the same position all day.

- Get enough sleep. If necessary, use an alarm clock to remind you that it is time *to go to bed*.

- Create order out of chaos. Organize your home and workspace so that you can always find the things you are looking for. Put things away where they belong, and you won't have to go through the panic and stress of looking for them when you need them.

- Take deep, slow breaths. When people feel stressed, they tend to breathe quickly and shallowly. This can lead to muscle tension due to inadequate oxidation of the tissues. Relax your muscles and take several deep breaths if you notice this happening to you. When you're relaxed, both your stomach and your chest expand when you breathe.

- Write down your feelings and thoughts in a journal or diary. Jotting your ideas and reflections down can sometimes help you see things more clearly and may even give you a new perspective on your life. Keep it out of reach of others so you don't have to worry about anyone reading your private thoughts.

- Use positive imaging to take the fear out of fearful events. For example, if you're going to be speaking before a large crowd and are afraid, go over every part of the experience in your mind in advance. Imagine what you'll wear, your walk to the podium, what the audience will be like, giving your speech, what the questions from the audience will be, and how you'll answer them. Visualize the way you would like everything to be. When the time comes for you to actually make the speech, the situation will seem more familiar and less threatening. Much of the anxious edge should have been removed by your positive mental imaging of the event.

- Give yourself a breather. Don't schedule your days so full that you don't have time to go to the bathroom. Back-to-back appointments are not always the best ways to get a job done. Allow yourself some time between appointments and avoid that harried feeling. Create a diversion for yourself between appointments with an exercise class or a walk outside.

- Discuss your problems with someone you trust, a friend or relative. This may clarify things in your mind and, at the very least, make you feel less alone.

- Try to avoid people and situations that cause you stress. Do people who gossip drive you mad? Don't sit next to Chatty Cathy at the next dinner party. Does talking on the phone for more than ten minutes set your teeth on edge? Hang up. Do you hate desk jobs? Don't take one—even if the pay *is* a little better than the nondesk job you were offered. Simple avoidance of the life-style and events that cause you stress can work wonders for your disposition and ward off headaches at the same time.

- Take a hot bath to relieve tension. (Try a cool one in the heat of the summer.)

- Do something to improve your appearance. Looking better can make you feel better too. Having your hair styled or getting a new suit or dress can give you the lift you need. Treat yourself right. As the commercial says, you're worth it.

- Eliminate self-destructive remarks like "I'm too old to . . ." or "I'm too fat to . . ."

- Make the most of weekends. Although you shouldn't alter your sleep patterns on weekends, a change of pace can do you good. If your weeks are normally hectic and filled with demands and people, use weekends to rest and be a recluse! If your work weeks are solitary affairs, socialize on weekends. If you sit all week in front of a computer terminal, get out and get some exercise on Saturdays and Sundays. If life is slow and predictable during the week, add adventure and spontaneity to your life on weekends.

• If an unpleasant task lies ahead of you, get it out of the way early in the morning so the rest of the day is anxiety-free.

• Don't be a do-it-all. Learn to delegate responsibility to others who are just as capable of getting the job done as you are. You needn't do it all yourself.

• Forgive and forget. Don't hold grudges. Accept the fact that the people around you and the world we live in are imperfect. Give other people the benefit of the doubt. Believe that most people are doing the best they can.

Learning to live with the natural stresses of life will help more than just your headaches. It should reward you with a new and healthier life-style. Besides following these stress-reducing tips, pay attention to good nutrition, regular exercise, and maintaining your good health. Be aware, as well, of the effects that your workplace environment and personal relationships have on you. Soon you will feel more in control of the stressful curves life throws you, and hopefully you will be better able to handle your headaches.

BIOFEEDBACK

Biofeedback can help you overcome your headaches because it teaches you to gain control of normally involuntary body functions such as heart rate, blood pressure, and muscle tension. Biofeedback has been used since the 1960s and has been proven very helpful in the treatment of certain headaches, especially migraines and tension headaches. In fact, some experts believe that with biofeedback training and relaxation therapy, nearly all tension headache sufferers can eliminate their headaches *and* more than half of those with migraines can avoid or abort their painful attacks!

Biofeedback teaches patients how to relax through electronic means. The process is painless, but it can take some time to master. About ten formal sessions plus practice at home are required. Follow-up sessions may also be suggested as a refresher course for later on. During the sessions, patients are attached to sophisticated electronic equipment. Sensors are placed on their skin to monitor their temperature, muscle tension, heart rate, and the like. One thing patients do is warm their hands, thereby diverting blood flow from the head. This temperature training has been very effective in reducing the severity and frequency of migraines. In electromyography (EMG) training, patients learn to recognize muscle tension in their foreheads, necks, shoulders, and jaws, and they learn to respond to that tension by deep relaxation (as in the relaxation exercises on pages 78–80). Biofeedback is also used in conjunction with visual imaging, which can have a physical effect on people that enables them to relax. Relaxation tapes can be listened to at home as well for continued relaxation practice. The National Headache Foundation has relaxation tapes available for order. Contact the foundation at 5252 North Western Avenue, Chicago, Illinois 60625. Or call 1-800-843-2256 (1-800-523-8858 within Illinois). In these ways patients learn to prevent headache attacks caused by overstimulation and overreaction to daily life.

These methods are most effective when practiced daily and used to prevent attacks. They are much less effective if a person waits until an attack is beginning and then tries to use them to abort it.

Interestingly, many patients who think they are relaxed are surprised when they receive feedback that shows they are not! It can be very difficult for some people to learn how to relax, especially after years of tension—which now seems to be the norm to them. Over time, however, almost anyone can master biofeedback techniques, as long as they attend all the sessions and practice daily at home. As they become proficient at relaxing, the reduction of their headaches becomes the most positive type of reinforcement.

Biofeedback will work for almost everyone, but it is not the answer to all headaches or illnesses. It will obviously have no effect on headaches caused by underlying pathological health problems such as brain tumors or eye disease. For this reason, we once again suggest that you do not attempt to diagnose and treat your own headaches.

ACUPUNCTURE

Acupuncture is now a much-talked-about remedy for many ailments, including headaches. As a method of pain treatment, it is several thousand years old and has been used most notably by the Chinese to prevent and cure health problems.

Acupuncture is performed with superfine stainless-steel needles, which are pricked into specific spots on the body and twirled or stimulated by electric current. There are between five hundred and eight hundred points on the body that an acupuncturist must know, and each one corresponds to a specific problem. For example, one point on the hand may be for toothaches while another may be for sore throats. The correct placement of needles supposedly balances the body's energy forces, thereby alleviating pain and disease, which are thought to be caused by an imbalance in the body. Electrical pulses in the needles may be used to enhance pain relief. Although all this may sound rather improbable, in certain situations acupuncture does seem to be an effective treatment. Headache relief (including migraine) may be one of those situations. The Chinese insist that acupuncture can work as an anesthetic and that surgery can be performed using only acupuncture as a pain killer.

How does acupuncture work? We don't really know. Some theories link it to the power of touch: A touch of the skin is, in fact, conducted along the nerves much more quickly than the sensation of pain. Touch can therefore override or block out painful stimuli in some cases. Other studies have suggested that acupuncture works because it causes the release of endogenous opiates, which can reduce pain.

Acupuncture treatment takes about twenty to thirty minutes, and several sessions may be necessary for maximum relief.

To find a practitioner, ask your doctor for a referral. Choose someone whose reputation is well known. If your doctor knows of no one, call a nearby medical university; they may be able to recommend someone. You can also try contacting a pain treatment center— your doctor or hospital may know of one in your area. But acupuncture remains a controversial treatment that has its advocates and its enemies. Before you turn to acupuncture, it is imperative that your headache pain be properly and accurately diagnosed. Doctors suggest that more conventional therapies be tried first.

TRANSCUTANEOUS ELECTRICAL
NERVE STIMULATION (TENS)

Transcutaneous electrical nerve stimulation (TENS) is theoretically somewhat similar to acupuncture in that it stimulates specific nerves to block out pain. Available by prescription since the early 1970s, it may counteract headache pain in some people.

The TENS device is a small, battery-powered pulsating stimulator about the size of a pack of cigarettes that can be worn under the clothing. The rate and strength of the pulses it emits can be controlled, and stimulation can be either periodic or continuous. The long-term success rate of TENS is variable. It seems to work best for localized pain affecting a small area and is believed to be about 50 percent effective. Although it appears to be safe, TENS is suggested for use in conjunction with other methods of pain relief. It has never been proven effective specifically for headaches.

HYPNOSIS

Hypnosis, the art of going into a hypnotic state, can help some people to control their headache pain. Specifically, hypnosis has been reported to provide relief from migraines. That headache pain may be controlled by hypnosis does not mean that the pain is all in the head to begin with. A hypnotic trance, rather, may simply block out physical pain. Hypnosis is therefore not a cure—it is only a tool for pain relief. The pain relief you achieve with it may be enough to enable you to get your life back on track, to regain control and set about finding real solutions to your headaches.

Unfortunately, hypnosis is not for everyone. Many people have great difficulty being hypnotized or learning to hypnotize themselves. Further, many people who can be hypnotized find that it doesn't help their pain very much, if at all. Very, very few people are able to block out pain entirely with hypnosis. Learning the art of self-hypnosis requires a skilled teacher, and these are not easy to find. Ask your doctor for the name of a professional skilled in the art of hypnosis. This person should be an M.D. or a Ph.D. whose reputation is well known to your doctor. Alternatively, a pain treatment center may have someone on staff who uses hypnosis. You can also call a nearby university hospital or medical school for a referral, or a local psychological society.

MENTAL IMAGERY

Most people daydream every day. They think back to a peaceful moment they enjoyed, rehearse something they want to say to someone, or relive the moment they got a raise. Such mental imagery can also purposefully be used to alleviate headaches. You may be able to escape the pain of a headache by deliberately "switching channels"—tuning out your headache and putting yourself into a relaxed and peaceful scene instead.

A psychologist can train you to use mental imagery to your advantage. He or she leads you through a pleasant memory and helps you recall the pleasant sights, sounds, and smells of that day on the beach or that fishing trip in the mountains. You and your therapist may even work together to make a tape of the daydream, reminding you of the things you see, hear, and smell along the way. You then listen to this tape and practice purposeful daydreaming. The goal is that when headache pain strikes, you can slip into this scene and take a "trip" lasting twenty minutes or so, from which you return refreshed and rested. Mental imagery may also be used as a relaxation method during stressful times to prevent headaches. Mental imagery is a way to give your mind a needed rest.

OTHER REMEDIES

Other, more offbeat remedies are currently under investigation and seem to work for some.

Sex is known to aggravate headaches in some people but has also been reported to help headache pain. In a Southern Illinois University School of Medicine study, one-quarter of female migraine sufferers found relief from headache pain through sex. Orgasm, they reported, could completely obliterate their headaches. Sex is thought to be beneficial because it diverts blood flow from the head.

For similar reasons, *hand-warming* also works for vascular headaches. In hand-warming, an accepted method of headache relief, patients bring the blood flow into their hands by imagining, for example, that their hands are in hot water. This technique can take some time to master and can be learned through biofeedback.

In *hot/cold therapy*, headache sufferers apply ice packs or heating pads to their necks and heads. Heat works to dilate blood vessels and may be of help to people suffering from tension headaches; massage of the neck and head also improves blood circulation to those areas. Cold can cause blood vessels to constrict and may be beneficial for vascular headaches.

Anecdotal observations have suggested other possible remedies, but hard proof or disproof is still years away. In a study at East Tennessee State University, for example, 100 to 200 milligrams of *magnesium* taken in pill form helped 70 percent of migraine sufferers overcome their migraines. This finding has not been confirmed by other studies, and more research is needed before such a remedy would gain widespread medical approval.

Another small study that has not yet gained universal medical approval points to *fatty fish oil* as a possible headache cure. The fish oil in question is EPA, or eicosapentanoic acid, which is found in salmon, mackerel, and other fatty fish. According to *Prevention* magazine, researchers at the University of Cincinnati College of Medicine found that the fish oil, taken over a six-week period, reduced the number of headaches experienced by eight migraine sufferers. The theory is that the oil reduces the release of serotonin and also may prevent blood vessel constriction. Migraine sufferers should not take this oil without a doctor's advice and supervision. Do not take fish oil capsules containing vitamins A or D, as the dose may be too high for you. Check with your physician first.

Feverfew, an herb, has been tried by headache sufferers for relief, but at present no one knows how much to take or whether these doses are safe or effective.

Remember, whether or not these nondrug methods work for you, you should continue to battle headache pain with all the resources available to you. If one method is not helpful, do not give up—try another. Eventually you will find a way, whether through nondrug methods or drug therapy, through pain treatment centers or headaches clinics, through doctors or psychologists. You *can* put headaches behind you.

NINE

HELP!
WHERE TO FIND IT,
HOW TO GET IT

Stop living with the pain, discomfort, and inconvenience of headaches. Help is available. There are many avenues that can be explored, from neurologists to psychiatrists, doctors' offices to hospital clinics. Unfortunately, many headache sufferers end up hopping from doctor to doctor, specialist to specialist, in their attempt to find relief from their pain. This chapter should prevent a lot of unnecessary switching and disappointments.

SEE YOUR OWN DOCTOR FIRST

If your symptoms are uncomplicated and not alarming, it may not be necessary for you to see a headache specialist. Your own doctor may be able to help you. It is certainly good to begin with him or her. Sadly, some doctors are not especially sympathetic to headache sufferers; others may mistakenly believe that if there is no underlying pathological *reason* for your headache, nothing can be done. Since only about 10 percent of headaches are caused by a serious underlying disorder, this would mean that about 90 percent of headache sufferers can't be helped! Not true—you can overcome your headaches.

Be equally wary of a doctor who prescribes medication for you without doing a complete workup, taking your history, or giving you a thorough physical exam. A doctor who is serious about getting to the root of your headache wants to know when your headaches first began, how frequent they are, how severe the pain is, whether you suffer from any associated symptoms, what factors trigger your headaches, where the pain is located, and which methods you have tried to relieve the pain.

If you find that your current doctor is not seriously searching for the root of your headache pain, you may want to consider switching doctors or turning to a specialist. Tell your current physician of your plans, and have your records forwarded to the new doctor. Finding the root of your headaches may be difficult, and hopping from doctor to doctor will not necessarily speed the process, so switch only if you feel it's really justified. Some patients feel that the ideal doctor is one who himself suffers from headaches, because he is likely to be more sympathetic and more aggressive in his exploration of causes and treatments.

If your regular doctor has difficulty unlocking the secrets of your pain or if he thinks a specialist should see you, he may suggest a headache specialist, a neurologist, a psychologist, and/or a psychiatrist. A neurologist is a medical doctor skilled in the treatment of the nervous system and nervous system diseases. This doctor has not only been through four years of medical school and three or four years of residency but has spent an additional two years or more on neurology as a specialty. A headache specialist may be a neurologist, internist, or otolaryngologist with a special interest in and experience with headaches. A psychiatrist (M.D.) or a psychologist (Ph.D.) might have a special interest in the treatment of headache and could help you with underlying emotional issues that may be related to your headaches.

To find a neurologist, psychiatrist, or other specialist:

1. Talk with your regular doctor about a referral. He will probably be able to recommend someone he trusts. In the unlikely event that he cannot give you a name or if you prefer to find your own specialist, read on.

2. Call a university hospital. Usually they can suggest a neurologist and/or psychiatrist. Ask if the hospital has a headache or pain clinic. This is often the best place to find the specialized help you need.

3. Get in touch with the National Headache Foundation (NHF). They may be able to help you locate someone in your area. Upon request, they will send you an extensive list of doctors who are members of the foundation and who have a special interest in the diagnosis and treatment of headache. The organization sponsors original headache research, especially on new treatments, and will also answer specific questions you may have about headaches. The NHF newsletter, published quarterly, is aimed at headache sufferers and provides information on the latest treatment and research. NHF is a membership organization. The annual fee is $15. Write them at: National Headache Foundation, 5252 North Western Avenue, Chicago, Illinois 60625 or call toll free 1-800-843-2256 (1-800-523-8858 within Illinois).

4. Go to the library and look under neurology and psychiatry in the *Directory of Medical Specialists*. Board-certified doctors are listed, with small biographies, by specialty.

5. Ask another headache sufferer for a recommendation. People in the same situation are often the best

sources. They can tell you who took their complaints seriously and who was able to help.

6. Check the list of headache clinics at the end of this chapter.

EYE DOCTORS

If eye disease is suspected or if you or your doctor thinks an eye exam would be a good idea, see a specialist for this. Many people are confused by the various eye specialities out there: This should help you to sort everyone out.

An *ophthalmologist* is a doctor with a specialty in eye disease. He can diagnose and treat problems and diseases of the eye and can perform eye surgery. An *optometrist* is not a doctor but a person skilled in prescribing glasses. He can measure the need for glasses and determine the necessary strength. (An ophthalmologist can also do this. An optometrist may in fact refer you to an ophthalmologist if you seem to have a problem other than poor eyesight.) An *optician* only fills the prescription. He sells and repairs the frames and makes eyeglasses to fit your specific prescription.

BIOFEEDBACK SPECIALISTS

If you decide to try biofeedback to help curb your headaches, you must find a qualified technician. Biofeedback is merely a technique—it must be applied by a registered biofeedback technician who understands the machinery. (Such technicians are not always doctors.) Finding the right specialist is sometimes a challenge. The Biofeedback Certification Institute of America in Wheat Ridge, Colorado, at telephone

(303) 420-2902, may be able to give you names of certified biofeedback technicians in your area. Ask for a
referral from your physician, a psychotherapist, psychiatrist, or psychoanalyst. Headache clinics often have
biofeedback technicians on staff. An M.D. or Ph.D.
with biofeedback experience need not be certified in biofeedback to be good. No matter who you choose, it's a
good idea to ask the person a few questions about their
training and credentials.

HEADACHE CLINICS

Headache clinics have recently been appearing across
the country. Such a clinic may be a good place to go
for help if you have been unable to receive a diagnosis
or get successful treatment from your regular physician. Usually they are devoted exclusively to the care
and treatment of headache patients. A headache clinic
is sometimes affiliated with a hospital and sometimes
not. It usually consists of a group of related medical
personnel, including staff neurologists, psychiatrists,
dentists, and biofeedback personnel. The personnel at
headache clinics are dedicated to persisting with the
problem and trying various therapies to bring your
headaches under control. This may take a great deal of
patience on the part of both the sufferer and the
personnel. It can take months of diagnosis and treatment, sometimes even years, before the most beneficial therapy is found.

Each patient should be dealt with on an individual
basis to find the root of the problem and the appropriate treatment plan. The treatments used at headache
clinics run the gamut from medications such as ergot-
amines, antidepressants, and calcium channel blockers
to nondrug methods such as biofeedback, sleep regula-

tion, special dietary plans, and if necessary, psychiatric help. Many headache clinics have facilities on the premises for such diagnostic tests as electrocardiograms (EKGs) and electroencephalograms (EEGs).

The headache clinic should be very thorough in its exams. On your first visit, your complete health and headache history will probably be taken. It may take an hour or more for your history to be completed, so thorough can the process be. After the history, the clinic will probably give you a complete neurological examination, including diagnostic tests such as blood chemistries, urinalysis, and EKGs. The multidisciplinary staff will then discuss diagnosis and treatment with you. Follow-up visits will be scheduled as well.

Various headache clinics that you can contact include:

CALIFORNIA

California Medical Clinic
  for Headache
19542 Ventura Boulevard
Encino, CA 91436
(818) 986-4248

Scripps Clinic and
  Research Foundation
10666 North Torrey Pines
  Road
La Jolla, CA 92037
(619) 455-8896

The San Francisco
  Headache Clinic
909 Hyde Street
Suite 230
San Francisco, CA 94109
(415) 673-4600

FLORIDA

Headache Management
  Center
1925 Mizell Avenue
Suite 100
Winter Park, FL 32792
(305) 628-2905

ILLINOIS

Diamond Headache
  Clinic
5252 North Western
  Avenue
Chicago, IL 60625
(312) 878-5558

KANSAS

Headache Clinic
Department of Neurology
University of Kansas
    Medical Center
39th and Rainbow
    Boulevard
Kansas City, KS 66103
(913) 588-6970

MARYLAND

Baltimore Headache
    Institute
11 East Chase Street
Suite 1A
Baltimore, MD 21202
(301) 547-0200

MASSACHUSETTS

The Headache Research
    Foundation
Faulkner Hospital
Allendale and Centre
    streets
Jamaica Plain, MA 02130
(617) 522-6969

MICHIGAN

Pain Clinic
University of Michigan
    Hospital
C-233 Med IMM Building
Box 0824
Ann Arbor, MI 48106
(313) 763-5459

MISSOURI

Pain Management Center
Menorah Medical Center
4949 Rockhill Road
Kansas City, MO 64110
(816) 276-8350

NEBRASKA

Midlands Neurological
    and Headache Center
401 East Gold Coast Road
Papillion, NE 68128
(402) 592-2611

NEW YORK

Headache Unit
Montefiore Medical
    Center
111 East 210 Street
Bronx, NY 10467
(212) 920-4203

Headache Clinic
Mount Sinai Hospital
Department of Ambulatory
    Care
Annenberg 3D
1 Gustave L. Levy Place
New York, NY 10029
(212) 241-7691

Elkind Headache Center
20 Archer Avenue
Mt. Vernon, NY 10550
(914) 667-2230

OHIO

TEXAS

Headache Department
Division of Internal
  Medicine
Cleveland Clinic
  Foundation
9500 Euclid Avenue
Cleveland, OH 44106
(216) 444-5654

Robert L. Hazelrigg, M.D.
4235 Secor
Toledo, OH 43623
(419) 473-3561

Houston Headache Clinic
1213 Hermann Drive
Suite 855
Houston, TX 77004
(713) 528-1916

John Stirling Meyer, M.D.
2940 Chevy Chase Drive
Houston, TX 77019
(713) 795-5807

PAIN TREATMENT CENTERS

At a pain treatment center, you will find a complete management team skilled in programs for mastering pain. Like the personnel at headache clinics, specialists from a number of different disciplines work together at pain treatment centers to diagnose and treat patients. A good pain treatment center pays attention to the "whole person" and does not concentrate on one technique only. Pain centers may be affiliated with hospitals or medical centers. Your regular doctor should be able to refer you to a reputable one. If not, check with a university hospital or medical school. Costs for treatment vary widely. Check to see whether your insurance covers any of these fees.

Obviously, pain treatment centers do not guarantee cures. Like all the other avenues you may pursue, this one may or may not work for you.

DIAGNOSTIC DILEMMAS

When you see a doctor for your headache pain, expect to receive a thorough and serious examination, including a detailed headache history. Be sure to tell the doctor what medications, if any, you currently take for your headache or other ailments. Mention any over-the-counter drugs that you frequently or currently use. (Pain killers that are used habitually may cease to be effective, and some researchers have suggested that the long-term use of analgesics can actually bring about the pain.)

HEADACHE HISTORY

Careful questioning on the doctor's part can lead to an accurate diagnosis, even in tricky cases. The doctor uses your headache history to search for a pattern and to try to pinpoint your headache type. Only when he knows what type of headache you have can he treat it properly. Your physician will ask you to:

- Describe your headaches. (The headache diary you completed in chapter 2 will help you answer this and the following questions.) If you suffer from more than one type of headache, be sure to explain this; do not omit to describe one type of headache in favor of another.

- Tell him at what age you began having headaches and when you began to have the type of headache you are now complaining of.

- Pinpoint the time of day or night when you are most likely to get a headache.

- Show him where the headache pain usually hits. It is important for diagnosis that your doctor know whether pain is generalized or occurs only on one side of the head. Citing a specific headache location, such as an eye, will help to narrow down the possibilities.

- Establish the frequency with which your headaches occur. Is it a daily or a weekly pain? Is it associated with your menstrual cycle? Does the headache appear only on vacations or weekends? Is it seasonal? Do the headaches appear for a time and then disappear for months?

- Indicate the duration of a typical headache attack. Does it come on suddenly and depart quickly? Do you suffer for hours or for days?

- Gauge the severity of the pain. Try to label the pain as severe, moderate, intense, boring, or the like. Use your own words to best describe the pain you feel.

- Tell him whether you experience a preheadache phase and, if so, what warning symptoms you experience. Do any disturbances of vision or speech precede your headaches?

- List any associated problems. If your nose runs or your eyes tear during the attacks, tell your doctor this. Do you experience nausea, light-headedness, or any other symptoms at the same time as your headaches?

• Tell him about any factors that seem to trigger your headaches, such as foods, menstruation, fatigue, tension, marital problems, vigorous exercise, bright sunlight, or alcohol. If menstruation seems to be a factor, the doctor will ask you further questions: Did your headaches disappear during pregnancy? Did menopause bring headache relief?

• Report whether your sleep has been affected—whether you have difficulty falling asleep at night or tend to wake up very early in the morning.

• Chronicle your family history of headaches. Does anyone else in your family suffer from headaches? If so, what type? You will be asked to give a complete family medical history, listing all other family illnesses as well.

• Detail any stressful emotional factors that may come into play. Are your home life, job, sex life, and social life all satisfactory to you, or do any of them disturb you or cause stress?

• Detail any environmental factors that may play a role in your headaches. Do you breathe in any unusual fumes at home or at work?

• Note any seasonal regularity to your headaches. Do they tend to bother you in the spring and fall? Do they seem worse around certain holidays? Do you experience seasonal allergies at the same time as your headaches?

• Report any accidents you may have had that caused trauma to your head. Even minor knocks should be mentioned just in case.

- List any recent medical information—your doctor will want to know about everything from a recent spinal tap or brain surgery to a history of seizures or tuberculosis. Any problems you have had with your eyes, ears, nose, or teeth should also be discussed at this time.

- Give him copies of any previous medical records that may bear on your headaches. If you have seen another physician for headaches, make sure your new doctor has all the information and the results of any tests that may have already been performed on you. Depending on when they were completed, there may be no need to repeat some of these tests.

- Tell him what medications you have already tried for your headaches. Which worked for you, and which didn't? What nondrug methods of treatment have you tried? Which, if any, worked for you? If you have allergies or sensitivities to any drugs, these should, of course, be mentioned.

- Tell him about any current medications you are taking for headaches or any other problem.

PHYSICAL AND NEUROLOGICAL EXAMINATIONS

Once the headache history has been taken and the doctor has asked you all the necessary questions, his next step will be to give you a complete physical examination (including weight, pulse, and blood pressure). This is usually accompanied by a neurological examination. Here are some of the things your doctor will be looking for as he goes about these exams.

General Observations

An observant doctor will, while chatting with you, pick up signs and signals that may help him in diagnosing your headache pain. For example, the doctor may notice signs of tension or depression while talking with you, or see signs of perfectionism if you are a migraine patient who unconsciously straightens up a few things in the doctor's office. Even certain facial characteristics may provide clues, as for cluster headache patients.

Physical Exams

The doctor will give you a thorough physical examination. He will probably check for high blood pressure, abnormalities of the spine, and bladder problems. Lab tests such as blood counts, blood chemistries, and urinalysis may also be performed to screen for diseases. Skull X rays, CAT scans, magnetic resonance imaging, and angiographic studies may also be ordered if indicated. Psychiatric testing may also be suggested if an emotional disturbance is suspected. Your head will be examined for any spots tender to the touch, evidence of local infection, sinus problems, or TMJ spasms. Muscle spasms in your back or reduced spinal mobility will be checked out. In an accompanying neurological exam, the specialist will check your coordination by watching you walk, stand on one foot, touch a finger to your nose, and catch a ball. Your reflexes will also be tested. The motor function of your trigeminal nerve will be tested by asking you to open your jaw against resistance. Your facial nerves will also be tested to see if they are functioning properly.

An eye examination should also be included. The doctor will look for vision problems, including possible glaucoma. A simple hearing test may also be done.

FURTHER TESTING

Sometimes the headache history and the general exams are not enough to diagnose. More tests may be needed for further investigation of headache pain. Such work may be called for if:

- The pain is chronic and persistent.

- Your headaches have not responded to various suggested therapies and medications.

- An organic disease is suspected.

- You have exertional headaches.

- You suffer from seizures.

- There is a change in type of headache you experience.

- Your headache does not fit a pattern and cannot be diagnosed.

Some doctors advise that skull X rays, CAT scans, magnetic resonance imaging (MRI), and/or EEGs be performed on almost all patients who complain of headache in order to rule out the remote possibility of organic diseases.

Whenever a doctor suggests a test, he should inform you of the reason for the test. You should also be told of any risks that may be associated with the test. For example, X rays carry the risks associated with radiation and are not advised for pregnant women. A spinal tap may cause a bad headache. At this time, the CAT scan and magnetic resonance imaging appear to be relatively risk-free procedures.

The following chart will help give you an idea of what tests may be used to diagnose which suspected problems.

Problem Suspected	Diagnostic Tests That May Be Used
general headache	physical examination
	headache history
	neurological examination
	electroencephalogram (EEG)
	skull X ray
	eye exam
	blood test
	CAT scan
	electromyography (EMG)
	magnetic resonance imaging (MRI)
migraine	all of the above
cluster	thermography
skull fracture	skull X ray
head injury	CAT scan
blood clot	CAT scan
tumor	MRI
meningitis	lumbar puncture (spinal tap)
brain disease	CAT scan

Problem Suspected	Diagnostic Tests That May Be Used
hydrocephalus	MRI
seizures	EEG
sinusitis	skull X ray
	MRI
	CAT scan
glaucoma	glaucoma test
stroke	angiogram
aneurysm	spinal tap
	CAT scan
	MRI
temporal arteritis	sedimentation rate (blood test)
	temporal artery biopsy
chronic facial pain due to TMJ	X rays of the temporomandibular joints
	dental examination
	MRI of the temporomandibular joints
spinal cord diseases	spine X ray
	EMG
	MRI

Here are some details on a few of these tests.

X rays

Skull and neck X rays may be taken. X rays show the bone but don't give a picture of what is going on in the brain. For this and other reasons, the plain X ray is being replaced by the more sophisticated CAT scan (see below). A plain X ray may show signs of a tumor indirectly, but a CAT scan or MRI shows it much more clearly and directly. An X ray will, however, show signs of skull injuries as well as deformities of the skull. X rays of the neck show arthritis, fractures, and other abnormalities. Sinus disease shows up in a sinus X ray. Pregnant women should avoid X rays unless they are absolutely necessary. Protective lead shields may be used to reduce the amount of radiation affecting other parts of the body.

Electroencephalogram (EEG)

The EEG provides a readout of the brain's electrical activity and patterns. During an EEG, the patient remains quiet while electrodes are attached to the scalp. Brain activity is translated into wavy lines that appear on a piece of paper and can be "read" by a qualified technician or doctor. The process is painless but may be slightly uncomfortable. The waves can show signs of epilepsy or even point to the unlikely presence of a brain tumor. They may help in the diagnosis of headache type.

CAT Scan or CT Scan (Computerized Axial Tomography)

A CAT scan is a highly sophisticated form of X ray. In a CAT scan of the brain, a very thin X-ray beam passes through a cross-section of the brain. Multiple measurements are made from many different angles, then transmitted to a computer through an electronic device called a scintillator. The computer reconstructs an image of the brain with black, gray, and white shaded areas that depict the bones, fluids, organs, and tissues. The image may be viewed on a screen or printed out. Each single scan requires only one to two seconds to take and involves less radiation exposure than a typical X ray. The average CAT scan might involve ten to fourteen scans of the head, and the whole process for the patient can take about a half hour.

Lumbar Puncture or Spinal Tap

The spinal tap is a test used to sample the fluid around the brain and spinal cord known as the cerebrospinal fluid. It can help in the diagnosis of several nervous system disorders, including meningitis infections and aneurysms. To perform the test, a small needle is placed in the lower back and spinal fluid is withdrawn. The patient either lies on his side in the fetal position or sits up and bends forward. The test may be uncomfortable but is not particularly painful. One side effect is that a few hours after the test, some patients get a headache. The CAT scan is currently replacing the spinal tap as the diagnostic tool of choice in many cases. Still, the spinal tap can be very important.

Cerebral Angiography

Cerebral angiography is essentially an X ray of the arterial blood vessels in the brain. Dye is injected into the neck to help outline arteries that cannot usually be seen in an X ray. A series of pictures are taken that show the circulation of the brain's blood. This test can reveal information about aneurysms that a CAT scan can't pick up. The test is also used to diagnose and define vascular malformations.

Electromyography (EMG)

Electromyography is performed to aid in the discovery of diseases affecting the muscles, spinal cord, and peripheral nerves. The test measures muscle activity in response to electrode or needle stimulation.

Magnetic Resonance Imaging (MRI)

The patient's body is placed in a strong magnetic field, and a cross-sectional image of the brain is reconstructed. The MRI process is much more complicated than that of the CAT scan. On the positive side, it involves no radiation, it is thought to be safe, and it gives the most accurate and detailed information about the soft tissues of the brain or other body parts. Some patients find the process uncomfortable, as they are placed in a tunnel for close to forty-five minutes; there they may feel isolated and hear a pounding noise made by the machine. Because of the magnetic field, patients with pacemakers and other sensitive electronic devices, certain clips, or other metal in their body cannot be given an MRI.

Even after all the tests are complete and the histories studied, the cause of headache pain sometimes remains elusive to diagnosis. Most of the time, however, a pattern is seen, a test confirms a suspicion, or a certain treatment has a beneficial effect.

Sometimes, very separate headache types can appear to be similar. For example, the difference between tension headaches and migraines, two such different head pains, can sometimes blur. Distinguishing a tension headache from a migraine is not always easy. Some symptoms that until recently were believed to be unique to tension headaches, such as the tensing of neck muscles, are now known to be just as common for migraine. Moreover, some of the statistics on migraine and tension headaches are quite similar: Both are more prevalent in women, both tend to run in families, and both have the same average age of onset. Some medical researchers now think that although the two headaches are different symptomatically, they may derive from the same neurological disorder. So be patient if diagnosis of your headache is slow in coming. Sometimes more time and more investigative work are needed to discover the true cause behind your headache.

In the meantime, however, continue searching for solutions to your headache problem. Your goal of a headache-free life should never be given up. Control of your headaches can be a reality. Continue to monitor your headaches, returning to the diary in chapter 2 if necessary. Try the various methods of headache avoidance and treatment mentioned in this book; turn to a specialist, headache center, or pain clinic if you are not finding relief elsewhere.

ELEVEN

EMOTIONAL MATTERS

If you are living with headaches that won't go away, you have to find ways to keep them from dominating and spoiling your private life, your work, and your family life.

Feeling sick is not easy. When you get headaches, you may feel sorry for yourself, angry that they are happening to you, and frightened that they might be a sign of underlying disease. By reading this book, by chronicling your headaches, and by seeing a doctor, you are taking the first steps toward gaining some control over these feelings and over your headaches.

Still, when you don't feel a hundred percent well, you're likely to expect more from your family and to place demands on them both emotionally and physically. When you suffer from headaches on a fairly regular basis, your family suffers too. Obviously what affects you affects them, albeit in a very different way. They may not be as compassionate as you'd like them to be. You cannot expect someone to send you a sympathy card for a migraine. In fact, even those close to you are probably not too happy to hear about your pain. They can't share it, and they may even suspect that you bring your pain on yourself. Seeing a doctor and getting an accurate diagnosis may quell their suspicions that there is something wrong with you emotionally.

In any case you may not get enough sympathy from your family. But look at things from their perspective. They cannot see your headache, the way they could see a cast on a broken arm. A child who finds that his dinner is not on the table does not feel sorry for Mom who is sick; he is much more likely to be upset that *his* needs aren't being met. All your family knows is how your illness affects *them*.

In fact, the average adult can run out of sympathy for an unwell family member in a matter of days. One spouse can mother another for only so long before he or she says, "A headache again. Oh, well—*my* life goes on." To avoid this dichotomy of interests, the family member with headaches has to remember to give back into the relationship what is taken out. Try to compensate your family members for their interest and help when you're down. Ask your spouse how the day was rather than complaining only about your own; make an effort to have food delivered when you're too sick to cook; praise a child who gets his own shoes on rather than bother you. When you're hurting with a headache, it can be really difficult to do these things. It's hard to think of anything besides your own pain at that point. But such efforts on your part reward your family and make them better able to give you love and support. It is important that you make an effort to relate to them.

If you need your spouse to do certain things for you when you're suffering from a headache, it's best to spell them out clearly beforehand. Just because you live together doesn't mean you can read each other's minds. If you need your spouse to put the kids to bed when you have a migraine, let him or her know. If you need him or her to watch TV in another room when you're having an attack, make it clear. If you think it will help, explain how the migraine affects you, that head movements, light, and sound are painful to you.

Your spouse may be happy to help you take preventive measures to control your headaches. Perhaps your spouse could help you practice your relaxation exercises by talking to you in a soothing tone or saying, "Relax your arm," and going through all the body parts with you. Your spouse can be a godsend if you find that massage helps your headache. Unfortunately, many husbands and wives are not so ready to give comfort, because they may not understand your pain. In a letter to *Prevention* magazine, a woman complained that her husband did not understand why "only a headache" could wipe her out the way it did.

If your relationship or your sense of self is suffering, you may want to find a psychiatrist or therapist to help you sort all this out. Do not be afraid to seek an expert. Your headaches may be caused in part by mental stress and conflict. Getting to the bottom of these problems could help end your headaches. Ask your doctor for a reference.

DENIAL

Some headache sufferers expend a lot of energy denying that they have a problem. Men in particular often believe that they are simply not supposed to get sick. A man with a headache may decide that it just won't stop him. A man may feel threatened by his headaches and fear that they will make him dependent on others. He will go to work half dead and expect a hero's burial.

Unfortunately, chronic or severe headaches occasionally *do* stop people, and headache sufferers have to face this fact. Do not put off treatment out of fear to admit weakness. If you put off dealing with your headaches, you are allowing them to control your life. Admit to yourself that something is wrong, find out as much as you can about your headaches, take active steps to prevent them, and seek professional help if necessary.

PARENTING

Children tend to automatically think that they are the cause of anything that goes wrong at home. If Mommy or Daddy is sick, a child may believe she did something to cause it. It's important to take your child off the hook. Let her know as plainly and clearly as you can that your illness has nothing to do with her behavior.

When possible, let your child know that you will be available for him later. For example, you might say, "I'm not feeling well right now, but I'll be able to read to you before bed tonight." It's fair to explain to the child that you're going to need his help from time to time—in the form of keeping the TV down or running an errand. When you have a headache, you may feel like shouting orders: "Shut that stereo off!" "Close the door!" Avoid commands; they rarely motivate people. Try to be gentle even when you're feeling murderous, and you'll get better results. Adding a "please" or a "would you mind" can go a long way toward eliciting cooperative behavior.

Give your children choices of how they can help. Say, "The shirts need to be picked up, and the garbage has to be taken out. Which can you get to today?"

Experts suggest that when children *do* help out, they should be rewarded. Depending on their age, you might want to give them a video to watch, some extra spending money, or just hugs and praise. *Do not bribe a child to do something,* however, as this can make the child feel used and resentful. There is a big difference between bribing and rewarding. On the positive side, your need for your children to help you during your occasional "down time" may make them more considerate people.

If you find that your pain occasionally makes it very difficult for you to keep your temper and cope with small children, step back from the situation. Leave the room. Get someone else to take over for you, if possible. Use deep breathing. Take a shower. Count to ten. Call a friend you can laugh with and get a new perspective on the situation.

THE ISSUE OF CONTROL

Even if you have used a pound of prevention, headaches may sometimes still strike you without warning. It can be hard to accept that even though you can control many of your headaches, you may not be able to banish them entirely. Some people react to this inability by putting extra pressure on themselves. They may feel that they must get three days' worth of work done in one day because tomorrow they may get a headache. This only adds to the very stress that can make your headaches worse.

Be kind to yourself. Resign yourself to the fact that "yes, I may get a headache tomorrow, but I have taken steps to guard against it, and that is all I can do." Accept the fact that you may occasionally have to succumb to a headache. Understand what you *can* control and what you *cannot,* and concentrate on the things you can control. For example, if you know that certain foods or sleep schedules trigger your headaches, feel good about exercising control in those areas. Don't waste energy fighting the fact that you sometimes get headaches. Work around them as best you can.

HEADACHES AND WORK

Obviously your headaches interfere with your work sometimes. Do the best you can to cope with this problem. First, seek help whenever a headache interferes with your ability to do your job. With the right diagnosis and treatment, you may be able to cut down significantly on the number and severity of your headache attacks. Use preventive measures to avoid headaches whenever possible: Leave your office for lunch, use deep breathing when things get tough, leave ten minutes early if you're really suffering. Although you may have to use the occasional sick day, don't make the whole office aware of all your problems. Try to keep talk of your malady to a minimum. It's unlikely that you will get sympathy in your office for not doing your work or not pulling your fair share.

DRUG DEPENDENCE

The risks of drug dependence for headache sufferers can be great. The drugs you take may be addictive. Make sure your doctor explains to you all the possible dangers and side effects when prescribing a drug. Don't con yourself into thinking that the over-the-counter medicines you self-prescribe are necessarily any safer or less addictive. Even aspirin can be overused and abused.

Occasionally, psychological factors lie at the root of drug dependence. Depression, anxiety, and insecurity can all lead to drug dependency. They are issues you can discuss with a professional. Get help for psychological troubles before drug addiction is added to your load of problems.

Sometimes people try to get attention by taking too many medications. They may believe that they will be ignored if they're well. When this happens to you or to a relative or friend, professional help is needed.

Some patients who become dependent on drugs end up hospitalized while they kick the habit. Remember, your goal is to prevent headaches, not to replace one health problem with another.

GLOSSARY

Abortive treatment: A remedy or therapy used after the headache has already begun. Taking aspirin for head pain, for example, is an abortive treatment.

Acetaminophen: An aspirin substitute. Like aspirin, acetaminophen works as a pain killer and fever reducer, but it does not produce the side effects associated with aspirin, such as stomach irritation.

Acupuncture: An ancient Chinese method of pain relief. Its effectiveness is a matter of some debate.

Allergy headache: A headache caused by a seasonal allergy and accompanied by watery eyes and nasal congestion.

Analgesic: A medication for pain relief. An analgesic works to increase the patient's pain threshold, thereby decreasing the sensation of pain. Analgesics range from aspirin and acetaminophen to narcotics.

Aneurysm: A weakened blood vessel. The vessel balloons out and may eventually rupture. In some cases, the rupture causes paralysis or death.

Arthritis: Inflammation of the joints, causing stiffness and pain in movement.

Biofeedback: A method of controlling normally automatic body functions such as muscle tension and hand temperature.

Caffeine withdrawal headache: A headache caused by dilation of the blood vessels once the constrictive effects of caffeine are no longer present.

CAT (computerized axial tomography) scan: A highly sophisticated X-ray technique for photographing the brain.

Cluster headache: A very severe headache; the pain is described as boring or searing. It usually affects only one side of the head, and although it is relatively short in duration, it recurs with some regularity over the course of a few days or weeks. It is then followed by an inactive phase, when the patient is headache free.

Electromyography (EMG): A test used to discover diseases of the muscles, spinal cord, and peripheral nerves. It can also be used therapeutically to teach patients when their muscles are contracting or relaxing.

Exertion headache: A headache that results from physical exertion, coughing, laughing, or sex. Its potentially serious causes demand immediate medical attention.

Glaucoma: An eye disease that can eventually cause blindness. Glaucoma is sometimes the cause of headache pain.

Hangover headache: A headache linked to the consumption of alcohol, which dilates and irritates the brain's blood vessels.

Hydrocephalus: An uncharacteristic swelling in the amount of cerebrospinal fluid within the skull, causing dangerous expansion of the cerebral ventricles.

Hypertension headache: A headache that strikes people who have very high blood pressure. Its "hatband"-type pain is most severe in the morning.

Hypoglycemia: A rare condition of low blood sugar, characterized by dizziness, sweating, and light-headedness. Hypoglycemia may be an early sign of diabetes.

Menstrual headache: A migrainelike headache that occurs with month-to-month regularity and is linked to the menstrual cycle.

Migraine: A vascular headache that usually strikes one side of the head or one spot, such as the eye. It is sometimes preceded by visual disturbances.

Neuralgia: The pain spasms of a major nerve. The pain is jabbing, sudden, and repetitive. There are several different types of neuralgias, and each affects a different area. Trigeminal neuralgia, for example, affects the nerves of the face.

Prodromal phase: The preheadache period of classic migraine, characterized by visual disturbances, speech disorders, and other signs.

Serotonin: A brain chemical that is believed to play a role in headaches.

Sinus headache: A headache caused by a clogged sinus cavity.

Sinusitis: An upper respiratory infection that blocks the sinuses, causing tenderness above and below the eyes and headache pain.

Temporal arteritis: A headache caused by inflamed arteries in the head and neck. It requires immediate medical attention.

Temporomandibular Joint Disorder (TMJ): A jaw disorder. It is sometimes linked to headache pain.

Tension headache: A headache characterized by tightness in the head and neck muscles. The pain is a generalized, dull ache.

Tic douloureux: A serious but rare disease of the neural impulses that mainly affects women over the age of fifty-five.

Trigeminal nerve: The fifth cranial nerve, a major nerve of the face and head. It is related to nerve impulses that direct the muscles for jaw movement.

Tumor headache: A headache caused by a tumor, or growth, that presses on the brain. Symptoms include seizures, loss of consciousness, projectile vomiting, and speech disturbances.

Vascular pain: Pain caused by the dilation or constriction of blood vessels. Dilating (enlarging) the blood vessels in the head causes pain when the vessels exert pressure on surrounding nerves. Constricting (narrowing) the blood vessels reduces the supply of blood to the brain. The tissue around the blood vessels may become inflamed, and chemical irritants build up in the area.

Vasoactive: Affecting the dilation or constriction of blood vessels.

INDEX

125